Step by Step
Trauma Management

Foreword

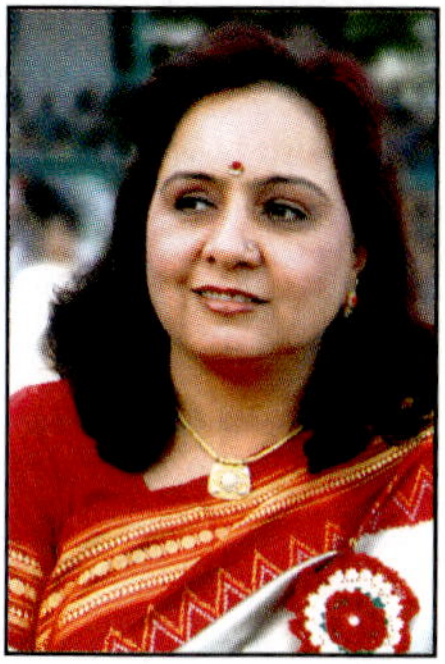

Trauma care is a daunting challenge because the golden hour, after a tragic accident or a sudden illness leads to the collapse of the human system in part or in toto, makes or mars life. Reaching out to the suffering in good time is in itself a task based on the response, i.e. time taken for an ambulance or anyone rushing help.

Even more important than that is handling the patient on hand with utmost care. Often, it goes unnoticed, that for want of proper handling the patient is put through greater suffering and, in some sad cases, lost life. To prevent the already bad condition from worsening a lot has to be done. Common misconceptions in providing immediate care have worked to the detriment of the trauma victim.

Fortunately, we are finally in an age and time when trauma care consortia are being grounded to rush immediate medical help in an emergency even as paramedics emerge as the first person of contact for substantive medical aid to victims. It is therefore imperative that paramedics and others who rush to help are fully conversant with what is to be done before expert medical attention is available. Both the paramedic and the health volunteer in the area of trauma care can benefit immensely from the following pages.

This concise and yet comprehensive manual by Dr. Chandra Bhushan and Dr. Chandra Sekhar Mone offers the commendable measures. They have explained in a simple and succinct manner what you may have to glean, in the normal course, by browsing through a medical encyclopaedia. Further, they explain vividly, with visuals, including illustrations, of remarkable clarity on what is to be done in the event of an injury or any other worsening health condition.

Seldom have medical professionals put together a utilitarian volume in this genre. The committed authors offer many lessons with which we can enrich ourselves, help prevent disabilities and save lives. Let us absorb and learn from it.

Mrs Tejdeep Kaur Menon
Deputy Commissioner of Police
Govt. of Andhra Pradesh

Preface

When we wanted to start a trauma care center at Global Hospitals in 2003, we realized that there were no paramedic training centers in Andhra Pradesh. Paramedic term was not well known in many of the hospitals in India. Prehospital care of the trauma patients was left to the bystander on the road or in its rudimentary stage.

We urgently had to formulate a syllabus and to train a group of youngsters to run our two wheeler ambulance services.

That is how this course material on step by step basis for trauma management by paramedic was formed. Throughout the course, the trainees used to attend the classes and work with us in the casualty for hands on training.

A handy Algorithm was developed for quick understanding and action by paramedics.

We believe that this book would be of use not only in the training of paramedics but also for a common man to get interested in the trauma care on the roads.

Chandra Bhushan
drcbhushan@yahoo.com
drcbhushan@gmail.com
Chandra Sekhar Mone
drcsmone58@yahoo.com

Acknowledgements

We sincerely thank the administration of Global Hospitals for giving us this opportunity to formulate the syllabus for paramedic training. Special thanks to Mr. D.R. Patnaik, Vice President, Business development, Dr. M. Veeraprasad, Vice President, Medical Services and Mr. K. Ramadar Naidu, Vice President at Global Hospitals for organizing the training for paramedics. The course material was used successfully to train groups of youngsters to become paramedics and get a career. This eventually led to the development of step by step book.

We thank our colleagues Dr. Hari Krishna, Dr. Sitaram Prasad, Dr. Subbaiah and Dr. PBN Gopal for their useful tips and material for the book.

We thank Jaypee Brothers for conducting the 1st Publisher Authors Meet at Hyderabad in 2004 for giving us enough stimulus to write this book and for promptly publishing this book.

Finally, we thank our family members for letting us spend our precious family time on working for the book.

Contents

Chapter 1

Introduction

A Paramedic by definition is a person trained in giving First Aid or Emergency medical care. Paramedics are usually deployed to take care of emergency pre-hospital medical care. They are also known as Emergency Medical Technicians (EMT).

The role of a Paramedic is very important. As time is precious in the care of a medical emergency, the availability, in time, of a trained, skilled and properly equipped paramedic is invaluable. He or She can deliver the same type of medical care as what would be expected in a standard hospital set up.

Injury (trauma) is the biggest killer of the young people aged below 40 years. Trauma is caused by road accidents, industrial accidents, natural calamities, riots, terrorism, etc. Every year eighty thousand trauma victims die and lacks of people are injured on the roads in India. The number of vehicles, plying on the roads, is increasing astronomically every year and the roads are getting congested. The number of road traffic accidents are increasing every year despite the widening of roads and imposing safety traffic regulations like wearing helmet and seat belts, speed restrictions, etc. Trauma is a serious medical and social problem of our society. Trauma is also called as a Neglected Disease of Modern Society.

In the west, it has been shown that high quality pre-hospital ambulance services and Specialized Trauma Centers can reduce the mortality rate by 400%. The key to this is the Golden Hour concept where the resuscitation measures have to be started in the first hour after the injury. This led to the development of Advanced Trauma Life Support (ATLS) system, by the American College of Surgeons, where doctors are trained for rapid assessment and resuscitation of trauma victims. This is accepted and practiced worldwide for treating trauma patients.

In India, we do not have a proper body or structure to deal with the large amount of trauma patients. Except for a few Metro cities, there is no organization to run high quality pre-hospital care ambulance services and trauma centers to treat the severely injured patients. We have the highest number of fatalities following automobile accidents in the world. Studies done by various organizations like the World Bank, National Academy of Sciences and the World Road Association have shown that the death rate is 2 people per thousand vehicles in USA and 140 people per thousand vehicles in India. The concept of Paramedics, who are trained, skilled and equipped, who can easily be made available at the site of accident at the earliest, is catching up in large cities. This involves lot of investment, infrastructure and management. In Andhra Pradesh, the government has started a unique Public–Private partnership scheme, called AP Emergency Medical Services, where a coordinated effort is called for from the Government Institutions like Director of Medical and Health Services, Major Government Hospitals and Private Corporate Hospitals. This was launched on 21st March 2004. The government has created a central coordinating office for accidents for the whole state with a single four-digit phone number 1056 and the major highways are adopted by the Corporate Hospitals to give Free First Aid to trauma victims on the road.

Global Hospitals, Hyderabad, has introduced a unique project consisting of ten Two–Wheeler Ambulances called Global Accident Rescue Team, G—ART. These two-wheeler ambulances are well equipped for immediate resuscitation of a trauma victim and also carry mobile phones for immediate communication. These are run by Paramedics who are trained at Global Hospitals. These two-wheeler ambulances keep roaming in the city in pre-selected routes. During heavy traffic times, these ambulances have been the first ones to reach at the accident site to start resuscitative measures on the trauma victims and mobilize them to the nearest Trauma center or Hospital. At many times, they have been at the accident site in less than five minutes (Figs 1.1A to C).

On 15th of August 2005, EMRI, Emergency Medical Research Institute was launched by Satyam Foundation in Public-Private Partnership with Government of AP with a three digit number 108. It has started with 30 Ambulance vehicles covering 5 cities in AP and plans to cover other parts of AP and also extend to other states.

This book is written as a part of the training structure for paramedics, keeping in view the Indian perspective. The objective is to make available a concise and compre-

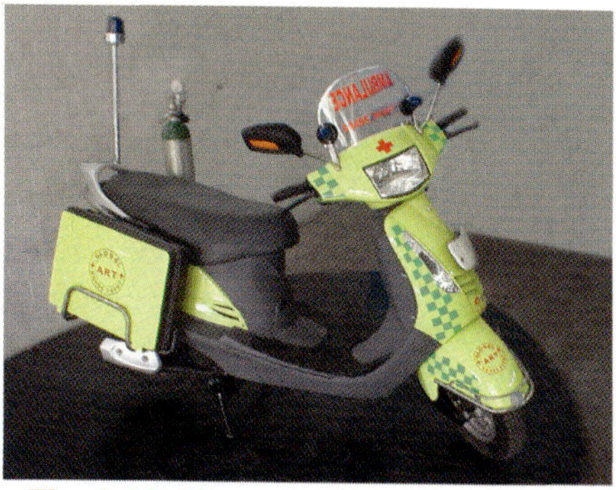

Fig. 1.1A: Two wheeler ambulance

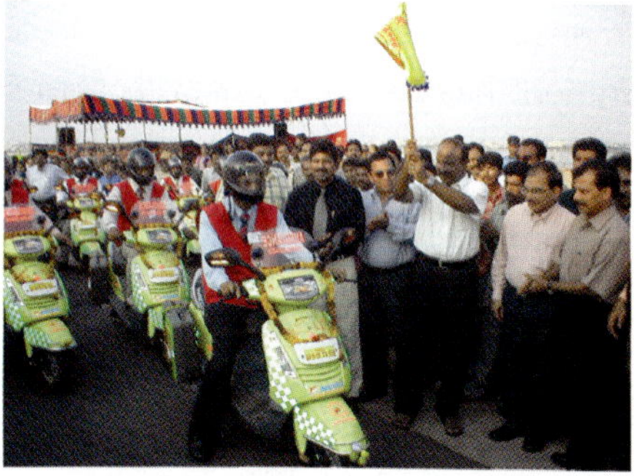

Fig. 1.1B: Flagging off G—ART

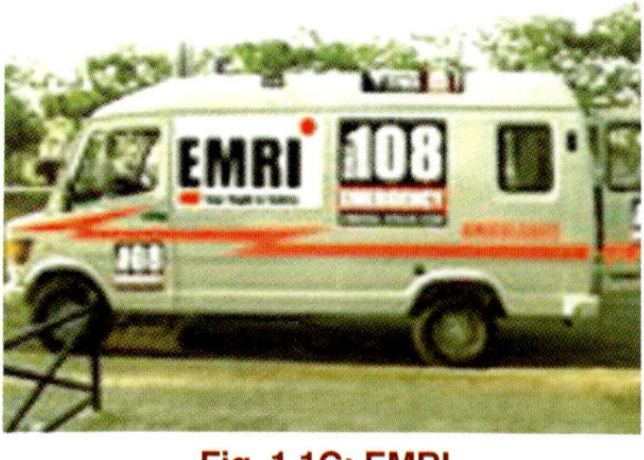

Fig. 1.1C: EMRI

hensive handbook with training program scheme. The book starts with a basic knowledge of Anatomy and Physiology of important systems of the body. Separate topics are included on Types of Injuries and Patient Evaluation at accident site. Special topics are given on Resuscitation and First Aid at the accident site. A handy Algorithm is included for quick management of a trauma victim. The Algorithm and Resuscitation are based on the principles of ATLS.

The awareness about the importance of paramedics in trauma management has to spread a lot in our country. The government has to come out with some legislation that all the ambulance drivers need to be Paramedics and that each major hospital in the cities and District General Hospitals should have at least six paramedics attached to casualty department (two per each 8 hour shift). More paramedic training centers need to be opened up. This way we can expect to raise the standards and efficiency of pre-hospital care of trauma patients.

Chapter 2

Human Anatomy and Physiology

RESPIRATORY SYSTEM

Structure (Fig. 2.1)

A. Upper airway (Upper respiratory tract): It consists of both nostrils mainly and partially mouth and these lead into one space behind the nostrils Called PHARYNX which descend down into voice box (Vocal cords).

B. Lower airway (Lower respiratory tract): It consists of trachea which starts below the Voice Box. The trachea descends down to bifurcate into two bronchi and each bronchus going into each right lung and left lung.

Later they divide into smaller bronchioles like that of a tree branches into the alveoli which are the primary areas for exchange of oxygen and carbon dioxide.

Oxygenation of blood is done in the alveoli.

Functions

Inspiration involves breathing in of air for oxygen and Expiration involves breathing out of air (Carbon dioxide).

Oxygenation of blood is very essential to the body and without which survival beyond 5-10 minutes is dangerous.

Normal Parameters

Respiratory Rate: 15–20 per minute.

Breathing in and out is heard by auscultation.

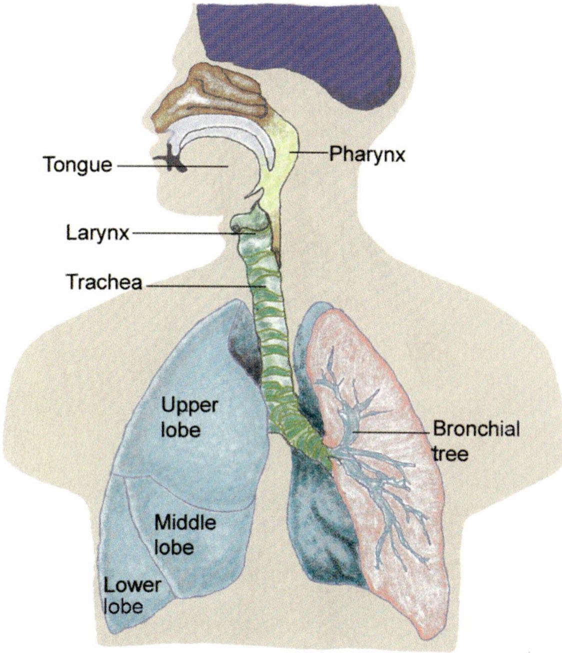

Fig. 2.1: Respiratory system

CARDIOVASCULAR SYSTEM

Structure (Figs 2.2 to 2.4)

- Heart
- Blood vessels—arteries and veins.
- Blood

  Heart—It consists of four chambers—right and left atrium and right and left ventricles. Right atrium receives the blood from the whole of the body and left atrium receives the blood from both the lungs.

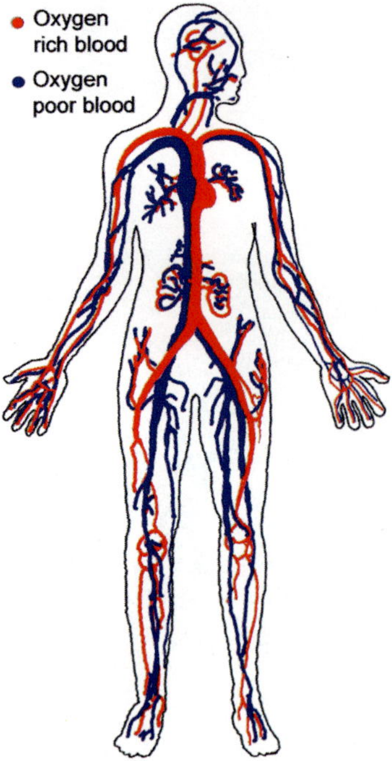

Fig. 2.2: Cardiovascular system

Right ventricle pumps blood from the heart to the lungs and left ventricle pumps the blood from heart to the whole of the body.

Blood consists of Red Blood Cells (RBC), White Blood Cells (WBC) and Plasma.

Functions

The heart beats and maintains the pressure in the vessels to supply the oxygen (carried in RBC) and important

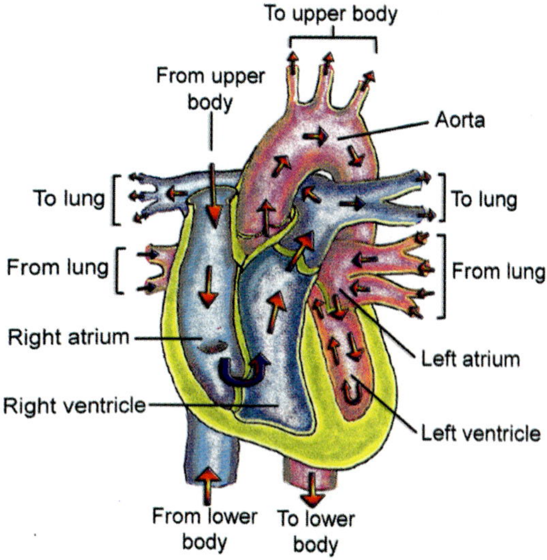

Fig. 2.3: Heart

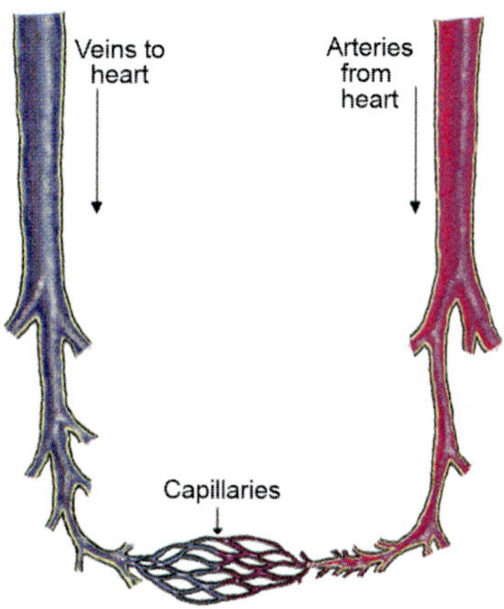

Fig. 2.4: Blood vessels

nutrients (carried in the Plasma) to the various tissues in the body.

Normal Parameters

The pulse is seen and felt at the wrist, neck and in the left side of the chest.

Pulse Rate: Average 80/minute

Blood Pressure (BP): 120/80 mm of Hg.

Heart Sounds heard by auscultation as Lub Dub.

GASTROINTESTINAL TRACT (GIT)

Structure

Consists of a long tract starting from lips through, mouth, pharynx, oesophagus, stomach, small intestines, large intestines, rectum and anal canal with its secretory organs like salivary glands, liver and pancreas (Fig. 2.5).

Functions

This is purely for digestion and absorption of swallowed food products.

Normal Parameters

Oral temperature 98.4°F.

URINARY SYSTEM

Structure

- Kidneys – 2
- Ureters – 2
- Bladder and Urethra

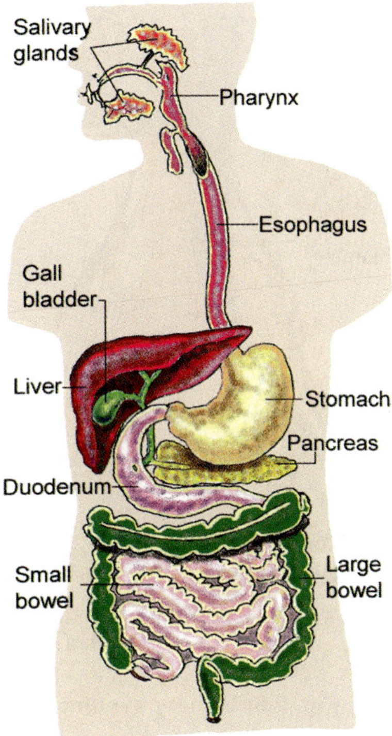

Fig. 2.5: Gastrointestinal system

Kidneys are located one on either side of vertebral column at about the Level of L1, L2 and L3 (Fig. 2.6).

Functions

Kidneys secrete urine by filtration of blood and pour into ureters and then into urinary bladder and later through urethra in external genitalia to be excreted out.

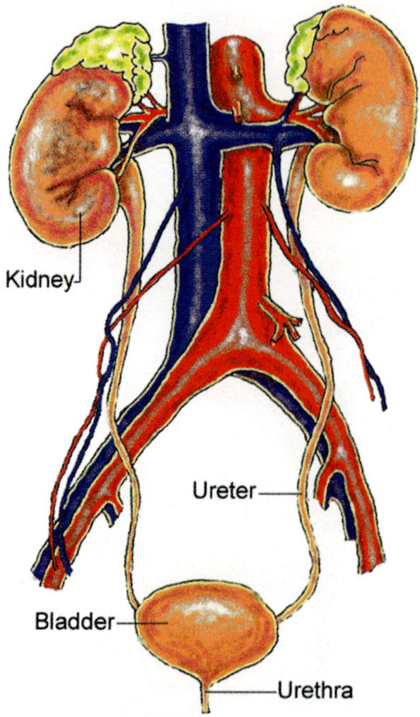

Fig. 2.6: Urinary system

Normal Parameters

Urine output of 1.5 to 2 liters per day.

NERVOUS SYSTEM

Structure

Brain, Brainstem, Spinal Cord and Nerves.

Brain and brainstem are located in the skull. The spinal cord is located in the spine along the back. And the nerves spread from the spinal cord to different parts of the body (Fig. 2.7A).

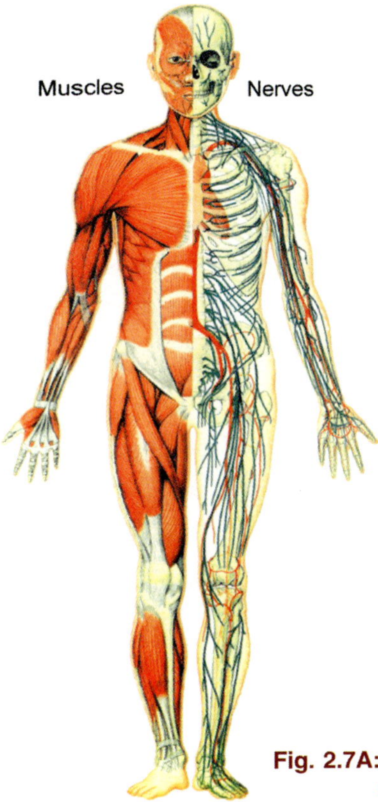

Fig. 2.7A: Neuro-musculo-skeletal system (Front)

Functions

Brain and brainstem act as the Consciousness Center and the Central controlling unit for all the functions of the body.

Spinal cord is like a Bundle of Wires leading to all parts of body carrying the different roles for motor power and crude sensations.

Normal Parameters

Consciousness, good motor power and full sensations.

MUSCULO-SKELETAL SYSTEM

Structure

Bones, Joints and Muscles.

The bulk of the mass in the limbs consists of bones and muscles. The joints are the junctions between bones for flexibility and movements. The muscles are the main contracting units for the power of movement (Fig. 2.7B).

Functions

Posture and stability of the body, locomotion and various movements of the body.

Normal Parameter

Ability to sit, stand and walk or movements of the limbs in bed.

SIMPLE CLINICAL METHODS

Signs of Life

Inspection

Consciousness—Verbal responses or Sounds.

Respiratory movements – Breathing – Respiratory rate.

- Observing the movements of chest.
- Feeling of movement of air on your finger, flowing through the Nostrils and Mouth

Eye opening and closure

Movements of limbs or body

Pulsations on left side of chest.

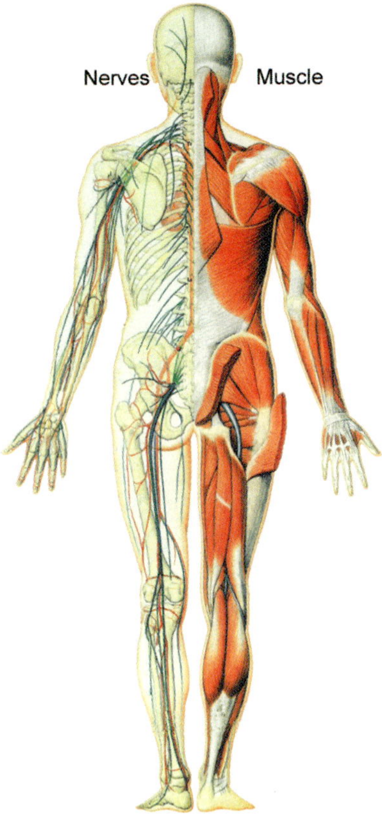

Fig. 2.7B: Neuro-musculo-skeletal system (Back)

Palpation and Maneuvers

Pulsations of important vessels at specific sites—Pulse Rate

Temperature of body, cold or still warm.

Pupils reaction to light

Auscultation of the respiratory sounds

Blood pressure measurement.

Chapter 3

Injury and Dynamics

TYPES OF INJURIES

A. Simple Injury

B. Complex Injury

C. Critical or Serious Injury

Simple Wounds

How to Identify

Patient is conscious and talking well and be able to go about if a little help is rendered whatever may be the wounds status either trivial fractures or minor wounds (Figs 3.1A and B).

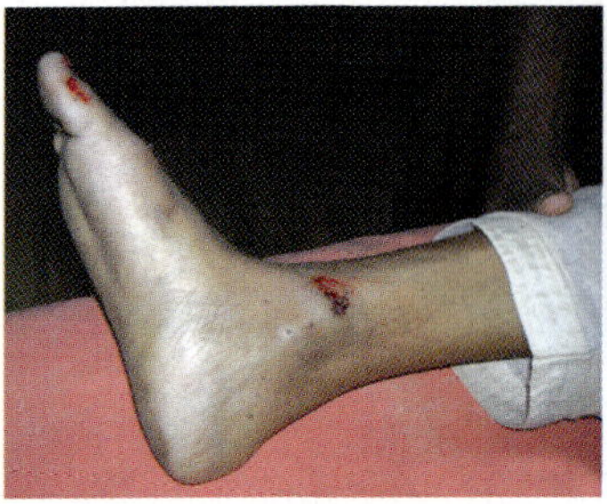

Fig. 3.1A: Simple wound—abrasions

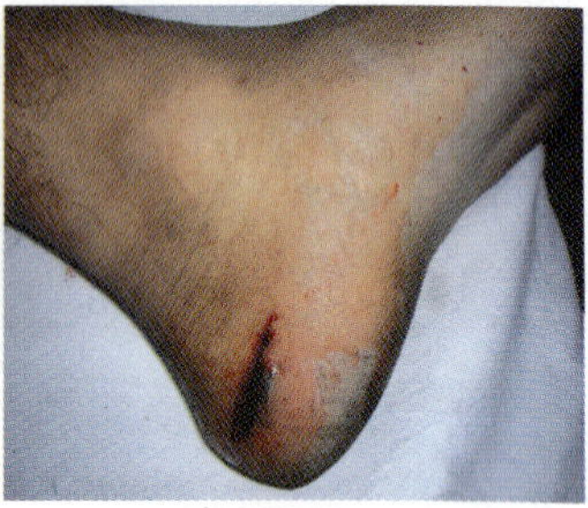

Fig. 3.1B: Simple wound—laceration

Mechanism

Direct injury with little force by a sharp or blunt object.

Examples

Simple scratch, Cuts or Lacerations, Bruising, Small Fractures, etc.

What to do

First Aid and Reassurance.

Complex Wounds

How to Identify

Patient is conscious with stable vitals but unable to move may be due to pain or due to injuries (Figs 3.2A and B).

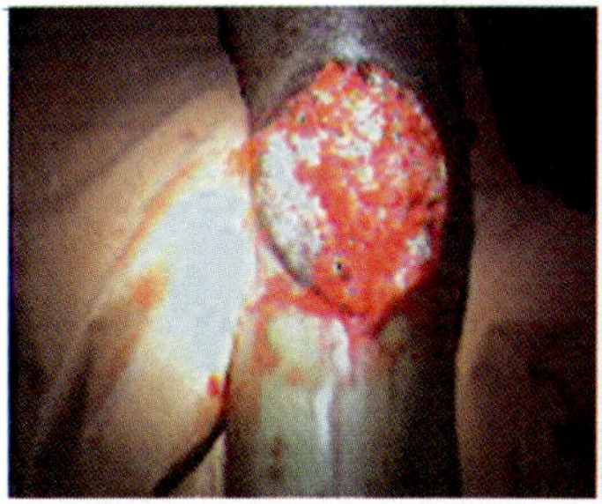

Fig. 3.2A: Complex wound 1

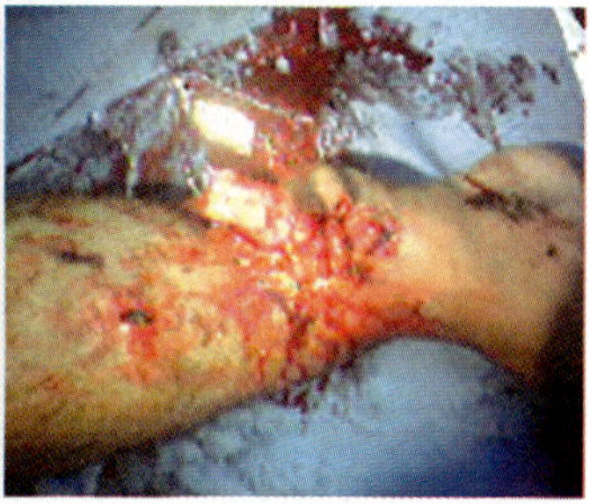

Fig. 3.2B: Complex wound 2

Mechanism

Direct injury with sharp or blunt object with more force or being caught between two surfaces.

Examples

Fractures of long bones, crush injury of a limb, closed head injury, blunt chest or abdomen injury, etc.

What to do

First Aid, Splint Application, IV Fluids and Quick Transfer to a Hospital.

Serious or Critical Wounds

How to Identify

Patient is not conscious and unable to move. Unstable vitals or in shock (Fig. 3.3).

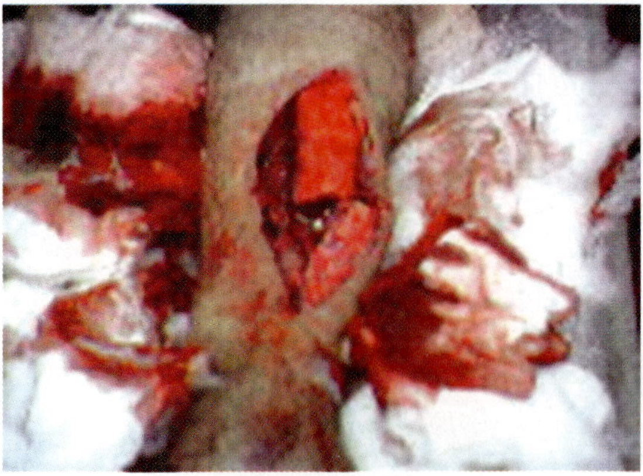

Fig. 3.3: Critical wound

Mechanism

Direct or indirect injury with severe force, being crushed between two surfaces or objects, etc.

Examples

Open or closed head injury (internal bleeding), open chest injury, open abdomen injury, severe crush injury of limb, etc.

What to do

Resuscitation, Oxygen, IV Fluids, First Aid, Splint Application, Immediate Transportation to a major Hospital.

SHOCK

Shock is an abnormal state of the patient.

How to Identify

- Low blood pressure
  - Systolic pressure is <100 mm and diastolic pressure is < 60 mm
- Increased Pulse Rate - >100 per minute
- Breathlessness – increased respiratory rate - > 30 per minute
- Skin – cold and pale
- Confusion, aggression, drowsiness and coma
- Thirst

Mechanism

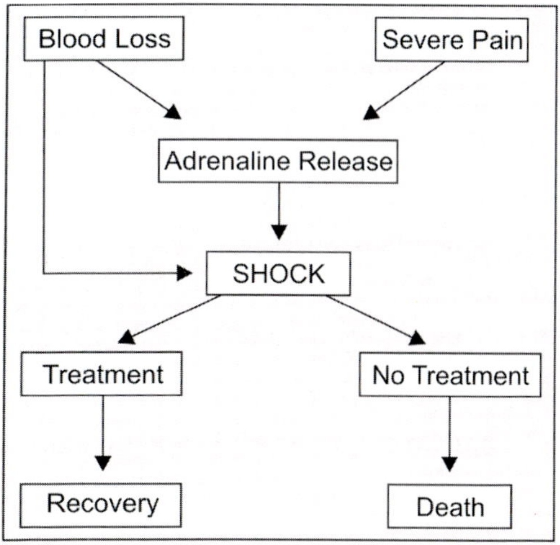

What to do

Resuscitation – Oxygen, IV fluids

Control of bleeding – Pressure, Dressings, Splints.

Blood transfusion

Pain killer (Analgesics)

HEAD INJURIES

Closed Head Injuries

An injury to head without any external wound.

Concussion

It is a transient loss of consciousness due to a closed head injury without any physical damage to brain tissue.

Examples: Acceleration and deceleration injury, direct mild blow, sudden shaking, etc.

What to do: Reassurance and to be sent to a nearby hospital.

Contusion

There is a localized damage to brain tissue due to a closed head injury (Fig. 3.4).

Patient may be conscious or unconscious and can have fits.

Examples: Direct blow on head, falling on side of head, etc.

What to do: If the patient is unconscious – give oxygen ventilation or resuscitation, Hard Cervical Collar and immediate transfer to a hospital.

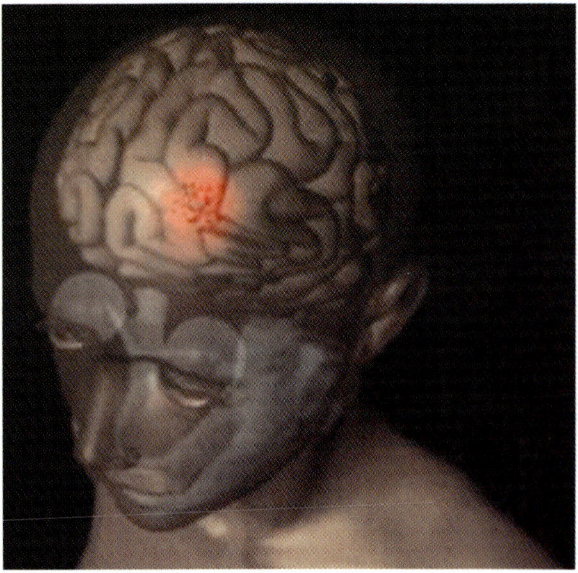

Fig. 3.4: Brain contusion

Hematoma

Extradural or intradural hematomas.

Patient can be conscious initially and gradually goes into unconscious state (Fig. 3.5).

Examples: Direct blow on head, falling on side of head, etc.

What to do: This cannot be diagnosed clinically, Hard Cervical Collar and should be sent to a hospital.

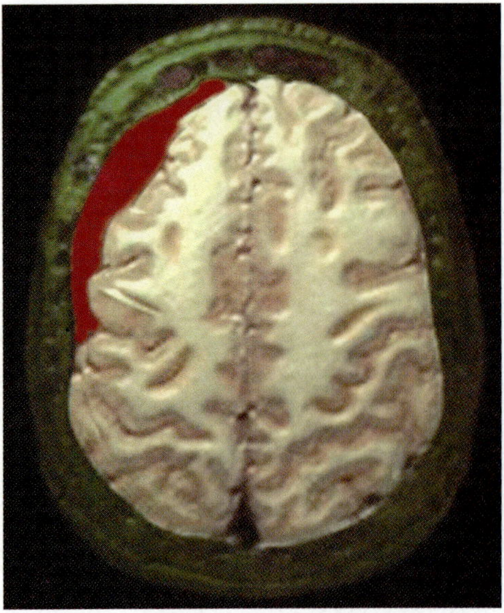

Fig. 3.5: Intracranial hematoma

Open Head Injuries

An injury to head with an external wound (Fig. 3.6).

Superficial Injury

Injury to scalp only and no skull or deep injury.

Examples: cuts or lacerations, avulsion of scalp, etc.

What to do: First Aid, Pressure to stop bleeding, send to a hospital.

Deep Injury

Injury to skull or brain tissue with an external wound. This results in fracture of the skull and damage to brain tissue.

Examples: Direct injury, crush injury, blast injury, etc.

What to do: Oxygen ventilation or resuscitation, Hard Cervical Collar, First aid and immediate transfer to a hospital.

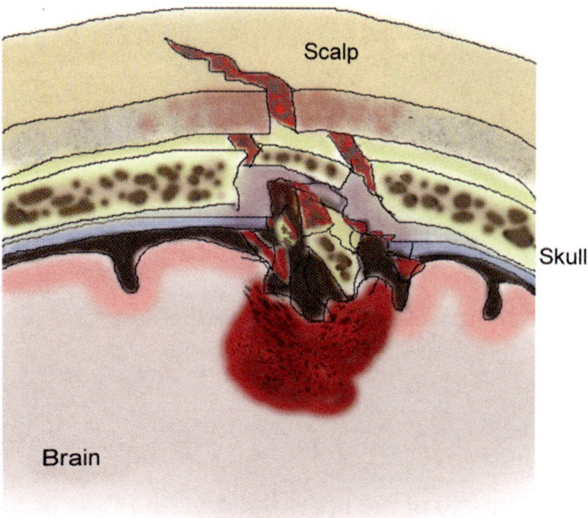

Fig. 3.6: Open head injury

FACIAL INJURIES

Facial injuries are common in Road Traffic Accidents. They may occur in isolation or in combination with other injuries. They pose problems because they are intimidating and obstruct access to the airway. Rarely they may cause life-threatening hemorrhage.

Injury to nose, mouth, eye, or ear may be present (Fig. 3.7).

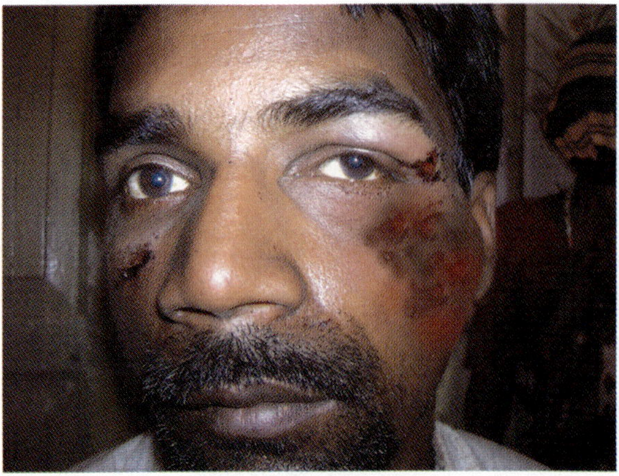

Fig. 3.7: Facial injury

What to do

The first priority of the resuscitation team is to secure and maintain an airway. This may involve going through an area littered with broken teeth and dentures, bits of fractured bone, and macerated soft tissue.

Clear the oral cavity by using a gloved finger inserted laterally (just inside the cheek) to the back of the mouth, then hook the finger medially and forward to pull the debris out of the mouth (If the finger is pushed centrally foreign bodies may be pushed further down the airway).

Repeat this maneuver from the opposite side of the mouth.

Use a large bore sucker to aspirate the oral cavity.

Airway.

Oxygen inhalation or Ambubag ventilation if required.

Stop bleeding by finger, thumb local pressure.

First aid dressings to wounds. (Avoid Betadine in the eye).

Shift to a hospital.

CHEST INJURIES

Many patients with catastrophic intrathoracic visceral injury such as laceration of the heart, aorta, or major airways die at the site of accident. In about 85% of chest injuries, the injury is confined to thoracic cage and underlying lung parenchyma (Fig. 3.8).

The basis for successful management of thoracic trauma is effective cardiopulmonary resuscitation followed by early detection and correction of life-threatening injuries.

Blunt Chest Injuries

Mechanisms and patterns of blunt thoracic trauma

Chest wall injuries	*Possible thoracic visceral injuries*	*Common associated injuries*
	High velocity impact (deceleration)	
Chest wall often intact or fractured sternum or bilateral rib fractures with anterior flail (caused by steering wheel)	Ruptured aorta Cardiac contusion Major airways injury Ruptured diaphragm	Head and facial injuries Fractured cervical spine Lacerated liver or spleen Long bone fractures
	Low velocity impact (direct blow)	
Lateral - Unilateral fractured ribs	Pulmonary contusion	Lacerated liver or spleen if ribs 6-12 are fractured
Anterior – fractured sternum	Cardiac contusion	
	Crush	
Antero-posterior–bilateral rib fractures with or without anterior flail	Ruptured bronchus Cardiac contusion	Fractured thoracic spine Lacerated liver or spleen
Lateral-ipsilateral fractures with or without flail Possible contra-lateral fractures	Pulmonary contusion	Lacerated liver or spleen

What to do

- Resuscitation
- Airway
- Oxygen inhalation or Ambubag ventilation
- IV fluids

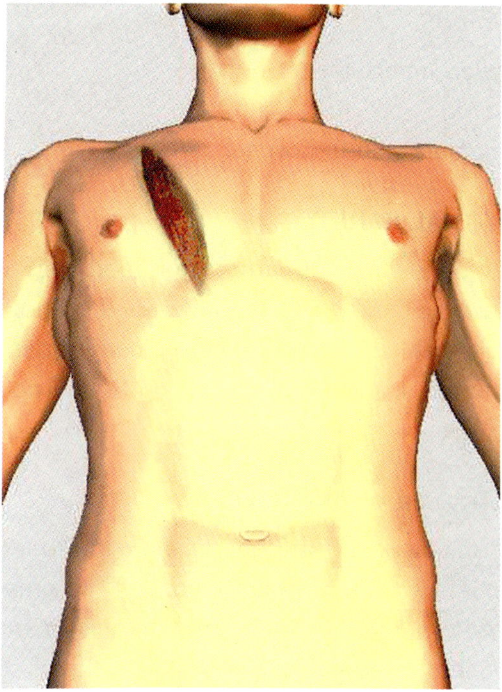

Fig. 3.8: Chest injury

- First Aid
- Immediate shift to hospital

Penetrating Injuries

Most penetrating wounds damage only the chest wall and the underlying lung.

When patients are seen with knives or transfixing implements still in place, no attempt should be made to remove these until the patient is seen by a surgeon.

What to do

- Oxygen inhalation
- First Aid
- Immediate shift to hospital.

ABDOMINAL INJURY

Intra-abdominal injuries carry a high morbidity and mortality because they are often not detected or their severity is underestimated. This is particularly common in cases of blunt trauma, in which there may be few or no external signs.

Blunt Trauma of Abdomen

Road traffic accidents are one of the commonest causes of blunt injuries. Since wearing seat belts was made compulsory the number of fatal head injuries has declined, but a pattern of blunt abdominal trauma that is specific to seat belt has emerged. This often includes avulsion injuries of the mesentery of the small bowel (Fig. 3.9).

The symptoms and signs of blunt abdominal trauma can be subtle, and consequently diagnosis is difficult.

A high degree of suspicion of underlying intra-abdominal injury must be adopted when dealing with blunt trauma.

Blunt abdominal trauma is usually associated with trauma to other areas, especially the head, chest and pelvis.

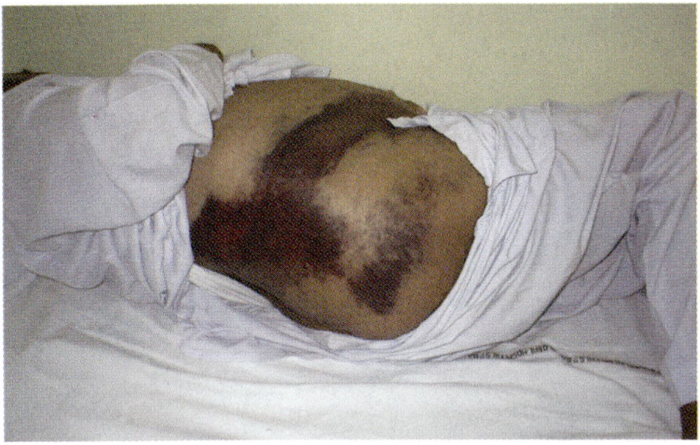

Fig. 3.9: Blunt injury abdomen

What to do

- Oxygen inhalation
- IV fluids
- Shift to hospital

Penetrating Trauma of Abdomen

Penetrating wounds are either due to low velocity projectiles such as knives or hand gun bullets or high velocity projectiles such as riffle bullets and shrapnel from bombs or blasts (Fig. 3.10).

Visceral injury occurs in 80-90% of bullet wounds but only 30% of stab wounds.

What to do

- Oxygen inhalation or Ambubag ventilation if required.
- IV fluids

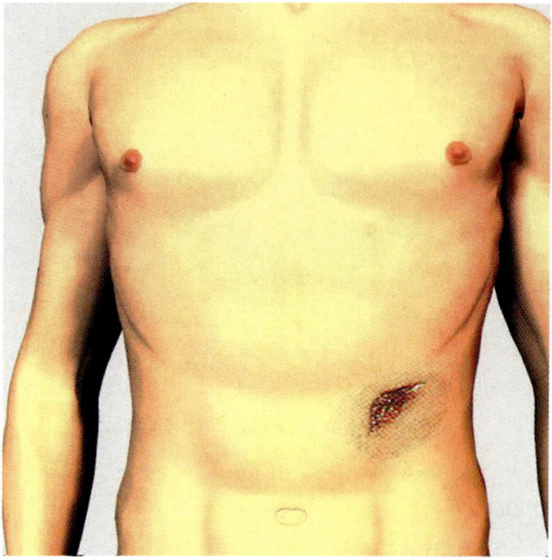

Fig. 3.10: Penetrating injury abdomen

- First Aid dressings to wounds
- Immediate shift to hospital.

URINARY TRACT INJURIES

Injuries of the abdomen result in injury to the upper urinary tract viz., kidney and ureter.

Injuries of the pelvis result in lower urinary tract viz., bladder and urethra.

Blunt Abdominal Injury

About 90% of renal injuries are caused by blunt abdominal trauma. A high index of suspicion of a renal lesion is required in the patient with multiple injuries as the signs and symptoms of the renal trauma may be obscured by those of the concomitant injuries (Fig. 3.11).

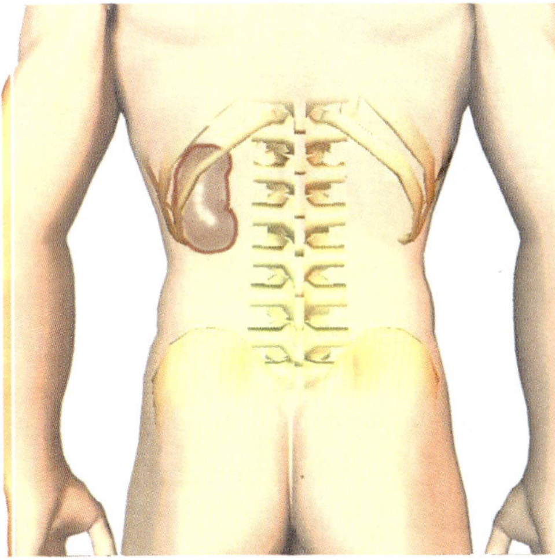

Fig. 3.11: Blunt injury to kidney

Direct injury: Sports injuries, run-over accidents and injuries caused by seat belts and steering column.

Indirect injury: Deceleration injury (falling from height and landing on buttocks).

Penetrating abdominal injury: Stab wounds, Gunshot wounds, etc.

Pelvic and perineal injuries: Crush injury of pelvis resulting in a fracture of pelvis can injure the bladder or inner part of urethra. A direct injury is like falling on to a bicycle crossbar or occasionally a penetrating injury (Fig. 3.12).

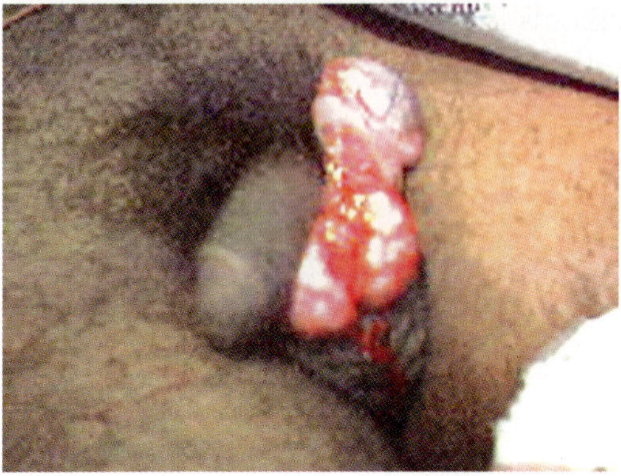

Fig. 3.12: Perineal injury – Evisceration of testes

Most patients (80-90%) with direct renal trauma give a history of a blow to the flank and complain of loin pain, which is followed by hematuria.

Examination shows skin abrasions or bruising overlying the upper abdomen, loin, or lower thoracic area.

Some of the patients can be in serious shock because of bleeding.

What to do

- Resuscitation with IV fluids
- First Aid dressings
- Shift to hospital.

SPINE INJURIES

Any patient with trauma who is not fully conscious should be assumed to have an injury of the cervical spine until proved otherwise.

A patient with serious multiple injuries is rarely able to provide a coherent history.

The commonest reason for failing to detect an important spinal injury is failure to suspect one, particularly in patients with multiple trauma; but sometimes a serious injury is considered minor.

The importance of spine injuries is its inherent element of spinal cord injury, which may result in permanent disability.

The injury to spine may vary from simple sprains to severe injuries like Fractures and Dislocations of bony elements of spine with or without damage to the spinal cord.

The injury to spinal cord may vary from simple transient concussion to partial injury, hemi-trans-section to complete trans-section of the cord with quadriplegia or paraplegia.

The spinal cord is most often damaged in the cervical region, but it is also particularly at risk near the thoracolumbar junction. Partial cord injuries are generally more common and the potential for neurological improvement or deterioration is correspondingly greater.

What to do

- Airway protection
- Oxygen inhalation
- Spine stabilization
- IV fluids
- Safe transfer to hospital.

Conscious Patient

The neck must be aligned in the neutral position without longitudinal compression or distraction. This will improve the airway and reduce spinal deformity, helping to relieve pressure on the spinal cord or arteries. Then apply the rigid Cervical Collar (Fig. 3.13).

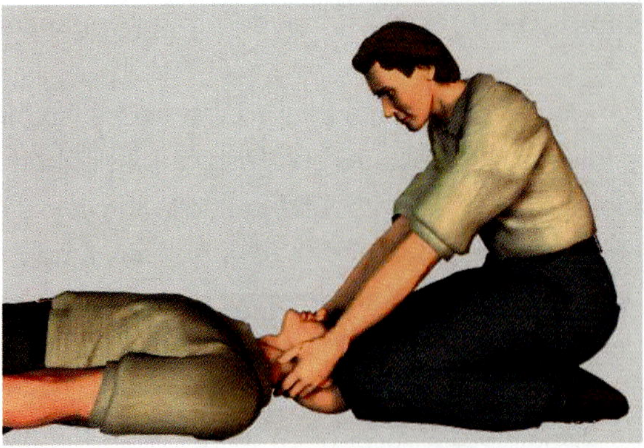

Fig. 3.13: Care of neck

Unconscious Patient

The airway should be opened by chin or jaw tilt and insert an oropharyngeal airway.

Keep the patient in supine position – good for CPR (if required), respiratory movements and control of neck, but endotracheal intubation is required to prevent aspiration (Fig. 3.14).

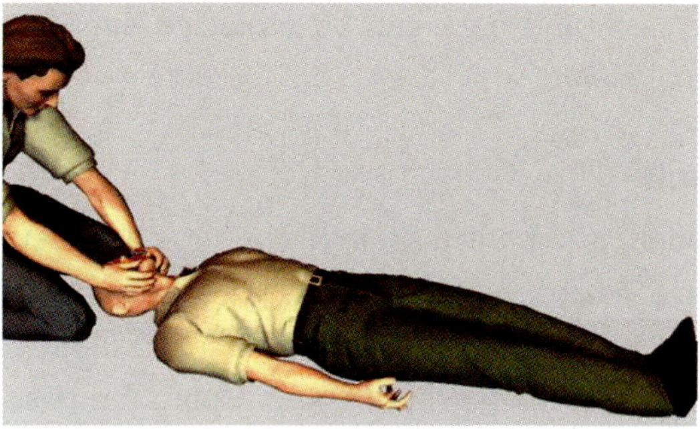

Fig. 3.14: Supine position with airway

Alternatively the patient can be turned into lateral position with the trunk straight but inclined forwards by 20 degrees, allowing secretions to discharge freely from the mouth (Fig. 3.15).

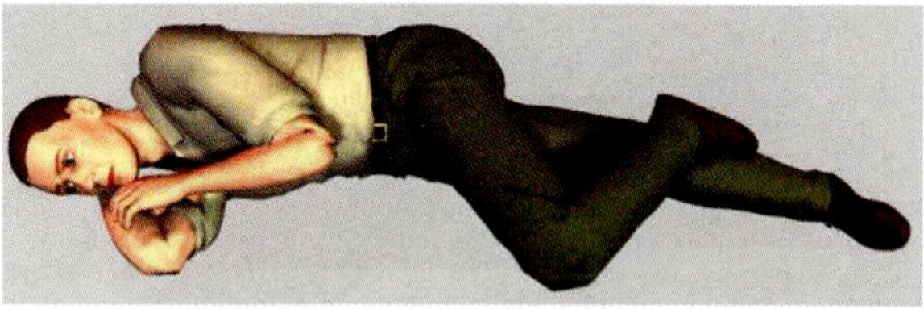

Fig. 3.15: Lateral recovery position

Thoracolumbar injury must also be assumed and treated by carefully straightening the trunk and correcting rotation. The patient may be log rolled or lifted as necessary (ideally by five assistants), but it is vital that the whole spine is maintained in the neutral position.

The neck and back can be protected simultaneously by Spinal Board.

Log Roll

The patient is log rolled on to his or her side, keeping the spine in the neutral position. This procedure requires 4–6 people and should be done as a synchronized movement. The person in-charge should be grasping the base of the neck and supporting the head with his or her wrists. If done correctly this is quite safe (Figs 3.16 and 3.17).

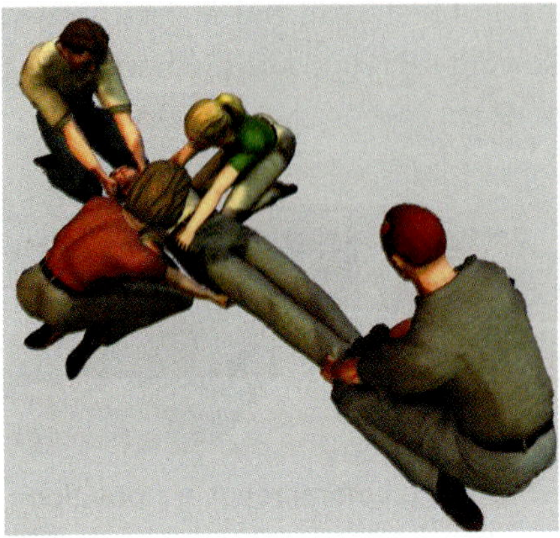

Fig. 3.16: Log roll 1

Log Lift

Safe transfer of the patient from the floor to stretcher or trolley can be done by 4-6 people, the person in-charge grasping the base of the neck and supporting the head

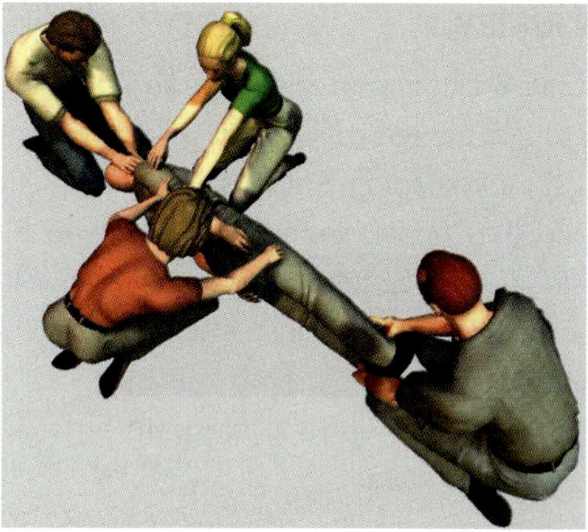

Fig. 3.17: Log roll 2

with his or her wrists. In this way there should be no seesaw movement of the neck (Fig. 3.18).

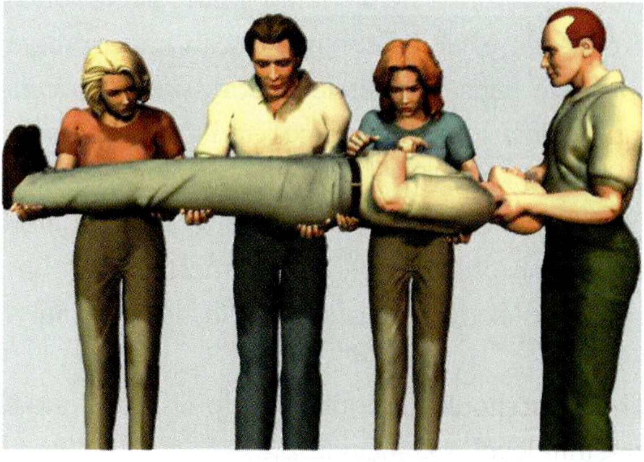

Fig. 3.18: Log lift

LIMB INJURIES

Limb injuries are common and occur in 70% of accidents. Resuscitation of the patient is of first priority as limb injuries are rarely life-threatening. Patients with multiple limb injuries can go into hypovolemic shock, due to blood loss from wounds and bleeding at fracture site, and they need to be transfused enough fluids. A rough rule of thumb is that a fracture in the upper limb can bleed up to 1 liter, one in the lower limb up to 2 liters and a pelvic fracture can bleed up to 3 liters.

When the patient with a fractured limb needs to be moved, the pain can be reduced by supporting the limb on either side of the fracture and applying gentle traction along the length of the limb. All unnecessary movements or handling of the injured limb should be avoided.

Wounds should be covered with sterile dressings. Severe bleeding can be controlled with finger pressure or compressive pads. Amputated parts should be collected in sterile saline soaked dressings and should be sent with the patient (Fig. 3.19).

Application of splints or support is a must before the transportation of the patient. Any material can be used for splinting like, wooden sticks, plastic or metal strips, etc.

The splint should immobilize the joint above and below the fracture level and include the bones on either side of a dislocation. The arm is supported by a simple sling. The

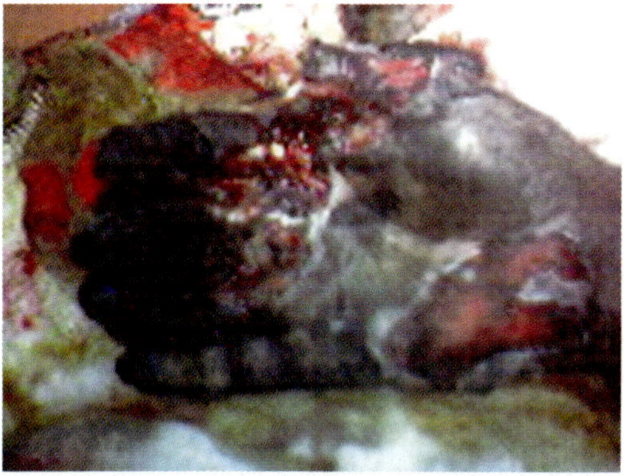

Fig. 3.19: Hand crush injury

forearm and wrist are immobilized by short padded splints or pillows. The leg and thigh should be immobilized by long padded splints (Fig. 3.20). Low pressure (30 mm Hg) inflatable double walled polyvinyl jacket splints can be used for immobilizing leg, ankle and forearm fractures.

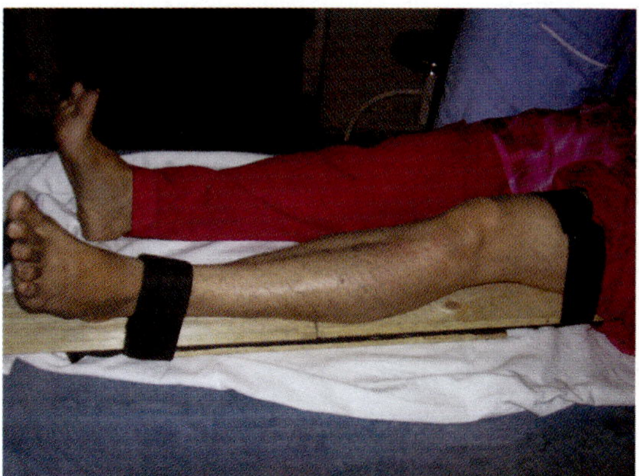

Fig. 3.20: Splint application

BURN INJURIES

Burn injuries are usually caused by industrial and kitchen accidents and sometimes by road accidents. Burn injuries can be of Thermal burns, Chemical burns or Electrical burns.

Burns are caused by dry heat, and scalds are caused by moist heat. Treatment is the same for both. The seriousness of the burn can be determined by its depth, extent, and location and by the age and the health of the casualty. Burns are classified according to their depth as first-degree, second-degree, and third-degree (Figs 3.21A to C).

First-degree Burns

First-degree burns involve only the first (epidermal) layer of the skin. The skin is red, dry, warm, sensitive to touch, and turns (blanches) white with pressure. Pain is mild to severe.

Second-degree Burns

Second-degree burns involve the first and part of the second (dermis) layer of the skin. The skin is red, blistered, weeping, and looks (spotted) mottled. Pain is moderate to severe, swelling often occurs.

Third-degree Burns

Third-degree burns involve all layers (full thickness) of the skin, penetrating into muscle, connective tissue, and bone. The skin may vary from white and lifeless to black and charred. Pain may be absent at the burn site. Third-degree burns are life-threatening.

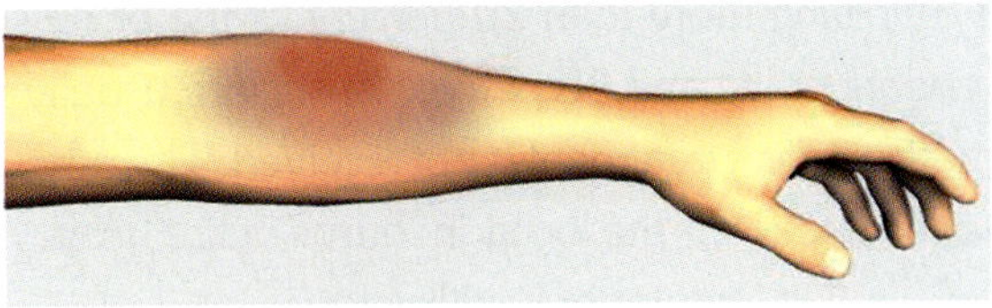

Fig. 3.21A: First-degree burn

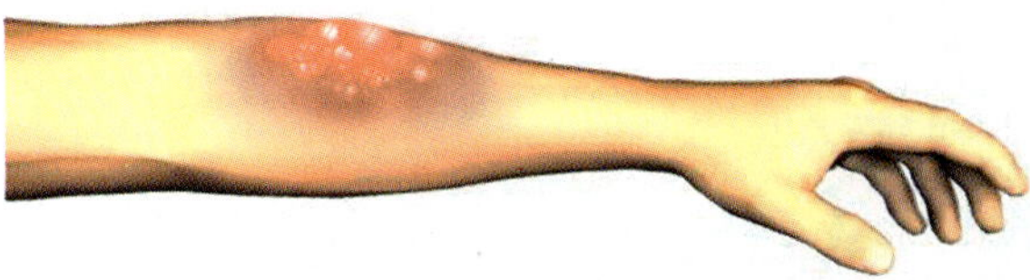

Fig. 3.21B: Second-degree burn

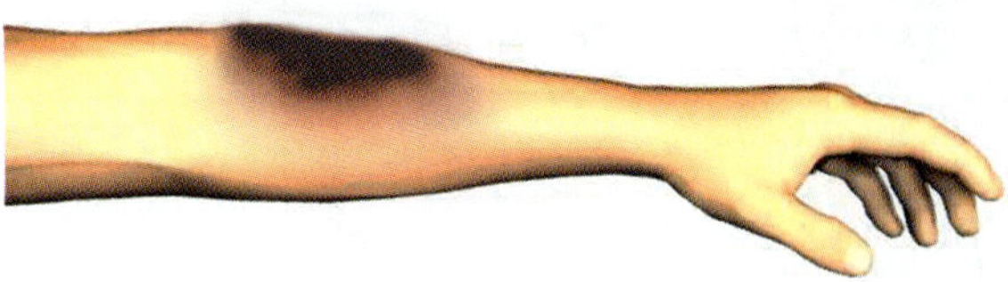

Fig. 3.21C: Third-degree burn

It is important to remember that the extent (size) of the burnt area is more important than the depth of the burn. A first-degree burn that covers a large area of the body is usually more serious than a small third-degree burn. The **"rule of nines"** is used to give a rough estimate of the surface area burned and aids in deciding the correct treatment (Fig. 3.22). Shock can be expected in adults with burns over 15 percent or in small children with burns over 10 percent of the body surface area (BSA). In adults, burns involving more than 20 percent of the body surface area endanger life and 30 percent burns are usually fatal if adequate medical treatment is not received. The other factor in burn evaluation is the location: burns of the head, hands, feet, or genitals require hospitalization.

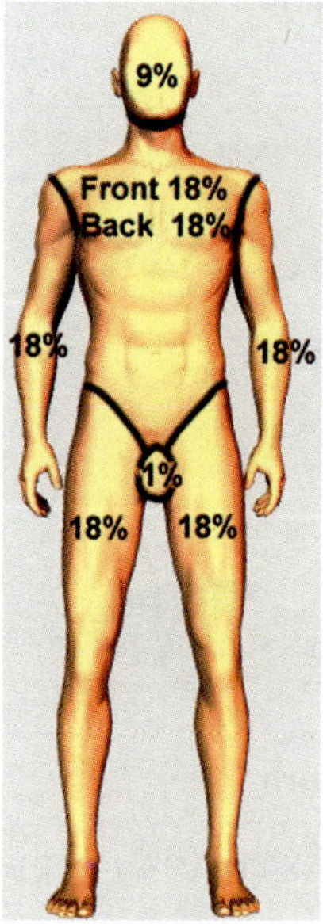

Fig. 3.22: Rule of nine

What to do:

ABC

Move the patient from the scene of injury to a place of safety and fresh air.

Give high flow **Oxygen inhalation** through face mask to all the patients with severe burns or exposed to smoke or fumes.

Remove all jewelry from the area. **Swelling may develop rapidly**.

Treat for shock. Give IV fluids (Normal saline) through a large size (14-16) IV cannula.

Cover area with dry, sterile dressings. Cover large areas with clean, dry sheets. **Do not break blisters or apply ointments of any kind**.

Thermal Burns

Apply cool water to the affected area or submerge in cool water. **Do not use ice or ice water**.

Remove clothing gently from the burned area. **Do not remove clothing that is sticking to the skin**.

Chemical Burns

Flush the area immediately with large quantities of fresh water, using a shower or hose, if available. Continue to flush the area for at least 15 minutes while removing the clothes, including shoes, socks, and jewelry.

Electrical Burns

Shut off the power

Cervical Collar

CPR

Chapter 4

Patient Evaluation

CONSCIOUSNESS

Consciousness is a state of normal cerebral activity in which the patient:

a. has awareness of himself and his environment

b. responds to changes in himself and environment.

Altered Consciousness

Sleep

As a normal variation in consciousness. Patient can arouse, either on his own or as response to external stimuli, to a full state of wakefulness.

Confusion state: Brain injury or disease.

Patient is alert but agitated, restless, frightened and disoriented in time, space and person.

Assessment

Assessment of level of consciousness is very important and will indicate the need for a change of management.

Abbreviated Coma Scale AVPU is useful in the initial assessment.

A = Alert

V = responds to Vocal stimuli

P = responds to Pain

U = Unresponsive (Coma)

Pain can be produced by pinching skin, squeezing Achilles tendon, sternal pressure applied with a hard blunt object or eyebrow pressure applied with a thumb.

Pupils

- Pupillary size and response to light should be noted.
- One pupil dilated: Intracranial hematoma
- Both pupils dilated: Raised intracranial pressure (ICP)
- Both pupils constricted (pinpoint pupils) and non-reacting: Pontine hemorrhage.
- Both Pupils Dilated and Non-Reacting: Brain death.

RESPIRATION

Respiration is one of the vital signs of the human body. The rate of respiration for a relaxed normal function adult is 14-18 breaths/minute.

The increased rate of respiration in an injured patient could be due to hypoxia or simple nervousness. Hypoxia can be due to airway obstruction, injury to chest (Lung or Heart), injury to brain or shock state.

Look: Movements of the chest

Feel: Feel with the back of the fingers, the movement of expired air from the nostrils or open mouth.

Listen: Listen for breath sounds on both sides of chest with stethoscope and ascertain whether they are equal on both sides.

Breath Sounds

Breath sounds are produced by the passage of air in and out of lung tissue. Normal (Vesicular) breathing is heard all over the chest, specially in the arm-pit and below the collar bone regions.

Throughout the inspiration, the sound is heard with a rustling quality and waves off in early expiration. Normally the inspiratory sound is heard for twice as long as the expiratory sound.

Care is taken that the chest piece (Stethoscope) is properly applied on the chest without undue pressure and not allowed to move or rub on the surface of the skin.

Breath sounds are absent in an area when their conduction is prevented by Pneumothorax (air in pleural cavity) or hemothorax (blood in pleural cavity).

PULSE

Pulse is one of the vital signs of the body.

Pulse is easily felt at one of the following sites:

Radial, Brachial, Carotid, Femoral, Posterior Tibial and Dorsalis Pedis (Figs 4.1A to C).

Features

The presence of pulse indicates the functioning of the heart.

Radial pulse at the wrist is generally used. It is felt with the tip of fingers.

The main features of the pulse are:

- Pulse rate
- Rhythm
- Volume

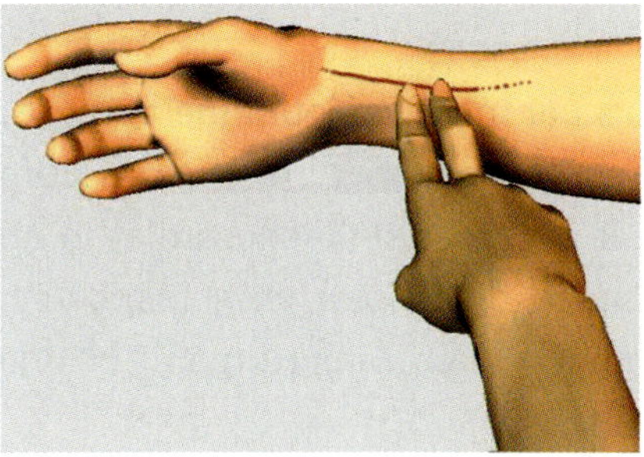

Fig. 4.1A: Radial pulse

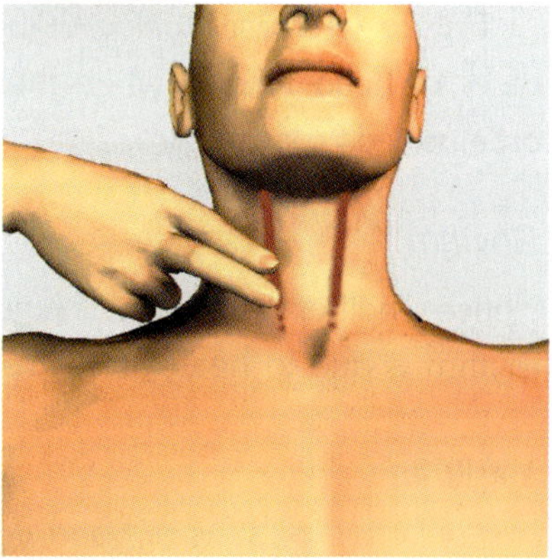

Fig. 4.1B: Carotid pulse

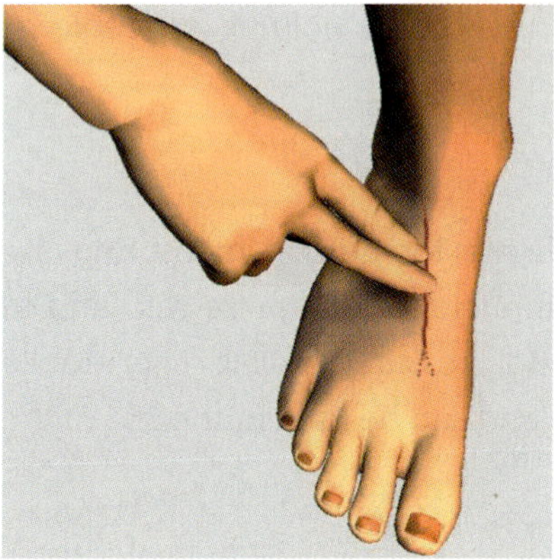

Fig. 4.1C: Dorsalis pedis pulse

Pulse Rate

It is the number of beats per minute. Count the beats for not less than half a minute. The normal rate varies from 60 to 100 per minute. It is increased (Tachycardia) in an accident victim due to shock (blood loss), chest injury with pressure on lungs or heart, stress of injury (pain) or due to simple nervousness.

Pulse is decreased below 60 beats per minute in certain cases of head injuries when there is hemorrhage in the brain, needs special care.

Rhythm

Notice whether the rhythm is regular or irregular. Irregular rhythm is due to heart problems.

Volume

Normally the pulse is of good volume and can easily be felt. In a shock patient, it is of low volume or feeble or difficult to feel it.

Pulse Oximeter

This is a very useful device for quickly measuring the oxygen saturation of peripheral blood, pulse rate and in some machines the blood pressure as well. The mobile machines are very small and can be used at the site of the accident (Fig. 4.2).

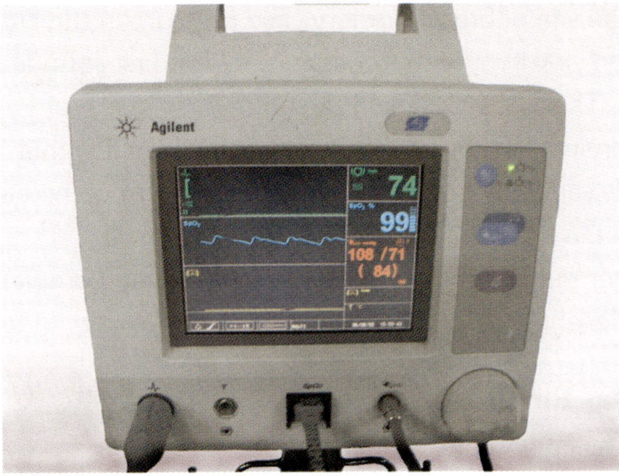

Fig. 4.2: Pulse oximeter

BLOOD PRESSURE

Blood pressure is one of the vital signs of the body. It roughly indicates the output of the heart.

Measurement

The patient could be sitting or lying at ease. All heavy clothing should be removed from the arm. The cuff should be applied closely to the upper arm, over the line brachial artery, with lower border of the cuff well above the elbow level. The site of brachial artery pulsation should be located.

The radial pulse is felt while the cuff is inflated to a pressure of 30 mm above the level at which the radial pulsation is no longer felt. The Stethoscope is then placed over the site of brachial artery. The pressure in the cuff is lowered slowly, 5 mm at a time, until the first sounds are heard. This is the Systolic Pressure.

Continue to lower the pressure in the cuff until the sounds suddenly become faint and disappear completely. This is the Diastolic Pressure.

After reading the pressure, deflate the cuff completely (zero level).

Normal Blood Pressure

In an healthy adult:

The systolic pressure is 100-140 mm Hg.

The diastolic pressure is 60-90 mm Hg.

In children, it is closer to the lower end of the range.

In elderly people, it reaches or even exceeds the higher figure.

The difference between the Systolic and the Diastolic pressures, the Pulse pressure, is 30-60 mm Hg.

In an accident victim, blood loss up to 1.5 liters will produce increased pulse rate (Tachycardia) and fall in pulse pressure, but the blood pressure may remain within normal limits.

A decreased Systolic pressure indicates that the victim has lost more than 1.5 liters of blood.

HEART SOUNDS

Heart sounds, one of the vital signs of life, indicate the functioning of heart.

Blood has to keep flowing in the vessels of the body for continuity of life. If blood stops flowing for more than 5 minutes to the brain, the brain tissue becomes dead and the person goes into coma. For continuity of blood flow, the heart has to keep pumping blood. It expands to fill with blood from veins and contracts to push the blood into the aorta and arteries.

Heart sounds are produced from the closure of the valves in the heart as the blood flows.

When the heart (ventricles) contracts, the Mitral and Tricuspid valves close down and produce the First Heart Sound (S1).

When the heart (ventricles) expands, the Aortic and Pulmonary valves close down and produce the Second Heart Sound (S2).

On auscultation, the heart sounds are classically described as LUB – DUB (S1–S2).

They are heard on the front side of the left chest.

Muffling of the heart sounds occurs in Hemopericardium or in the thick chest wall.

BLEEDING

Blood flows in a closed cardiovascular system. Bleeding is leakage or flowing of blood out of the closed cardio-vascular system.

Types of Bleeding

1. External – Bleeding out of the body or surface. It is evident.
2. Internal – Bleeding either into muscle planes and under the skin as in fractures or intraluminal as in abdominal or chest injuries. The signs are swelling, distention, echemosis, discomfort, tenderness.

A. Capillary bleeding – as at fingertip bleeding. It is slow and little and stops on its own.

B. Venous bleeding – can ooze to a good volume and stops on pressure application. Bleeding from large veins can be dangerous.

C. Arterial bleeding – is dangerous. It can bleed fast and can lead to shock and then death. Bleeding is in spurts along with pulsations. Sometimes the cut artery goes into spasm and stops the bleeding on its own.

What to do

Any external bleeding can be stopped with local pressure. Put a thumb or a finger and maintain pressure constantly without shaking or movement for 3-5 minutes for the formation of blood clot. And release the pressure slowly.

If the bleeding is from a large vessel – pressure has to be maintained till the patient is taken to a hospital.

VOMITING

Vomiting in a trauma patient occurs due to:

1. Injury to abdomen

2. Injury to head (raised intracranial pressure—ICP)
3. Swallowing of blood
4. Neurogenic shock like status due to trauma
5. Simple trauma nervousness in a patient with full stomach.

Vomiting in an unconscious patient has to be taken care of. The head should be lowered and face to be turned to one side for the flow of the contents, to avoid aspiration of the contents into the lungs. Suction should be used to clear the mouth and nose for free airway clearance.

SIT, STAND AND WALK

Sitting up, Standing and Walking involve lot of coordination of different systems of the body.

They involve proper functioning of:

1. *Musculo-skeletal system:* consisting of bones, joints, muscles and ligaments.
2. *Peripheral nervous system:* consisting of several nerves to various parts of the trunk and limbs – for carrying motor signals to muscles, sensory signals from various sense organs from skin and proprioceptive signals from joints.
3. *Central nervous system (several parts of brain and spinal cord):* for balancing, coordination, understanding, orientation, etc.
4. *Visual system:* with eyes, orbital muscles, optic nerve and brain – for coordination and orientation.
5. *Auditory system:* consisting of ears, and vestibules for Orientation, balancing, etc.

When a person obeys your command and is able to sit up, stand and walk, then the above given systems can quickly and grossly be considered to be normal. This is useful in disaster management when you need to identify the more critical patients among several accident victims by doing quick examination without wasting critical time.

LIMB MOVEMENTS

When the patient is not able to sit up, stand and is walk or not supposed to do so (head injury, neck injury, spine injury), we can do a quick assessment of the limbs for any serious injury.

Upper Limb

If the patient is able to make a fist with the hand and open all the fingers, able to feel all the fingers, flex and extend the elbow, and lift up the limb up in air from the shoulder – then there is no major injury to the limb.

Lower Limb

If the patient is able to feel all the toes, able to move the foot up and down, flex and extend the knee and able to lift the limb up in air from the hip – then there is no major injury to the limb.

Chapter 5

Resuscitation

ABCD

Airway

Assessment: any signs of obstruction?

Ascertain patency

Management; establish a patent airway

Protect cervical spine.

Breathing

Assessment: determine respiratory rate, check bilateral chest movements, percuss and auscultate.

Management: If no respiratory effort, treat as arrest. If breathing is compromised, give high concentration of Oxygen, manage according to findings, e.g. relieve tension pneumothorax.

Circulation

Assessment: check pulse and BP, is he/she peripherally shut down? Look for evidence of bleeding.

Management: If no cardiac output, treat it as arrest. If shocked, treat with IV fluids, oxygen.

Disability

Assessment: level of consciousness – AVPU

Pupils – size, whether equal and reactive.

Limb deformities and disabilities.

AIRWAY CLEARANCE

This is of utmost importance. This is one of the simplest measures and should be done very quickly as soon as you approach the patient.

Ask the patient his/her name or any question. If the patient responds with a normal voice and gives logical answers to your questions, the airway is patent and the brain is functioning properly.

If there is no reply from the patient, open the patient's mouth and remove any blood, liquid vomit, etc. with a sucker. Remove false teeth and any other solid foreign object with forceps or fingers. Lift the chin up, depress the tongue and put in an airway. Give 100% Oxygen ventilation (Figs 5.1A to C).

Caution: In an unconscious patient, consider the neck (cervical spine). Is it broken or dislocated? It is very important not to make the patient worse by your manipulations.

It is better to stabilize it by cervical collar.

OXYGEN INHALATION/VENTILATION

All severely injured patients should be given oxygen. Make sure the airway is free and breathing is unimpaired. Count the respiratory rate and see the depth of breathing and exertion for breathing.

If the patient is breathing well with or without exertion and a free airway, give oxygen inhalation with a face mask.

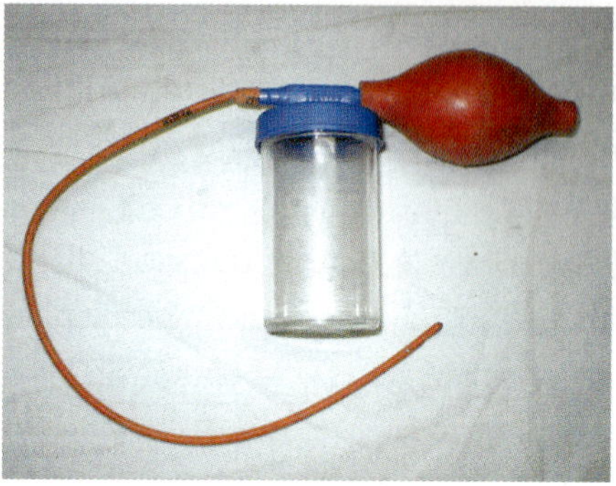

Fig. 5.1A: Hand sucker

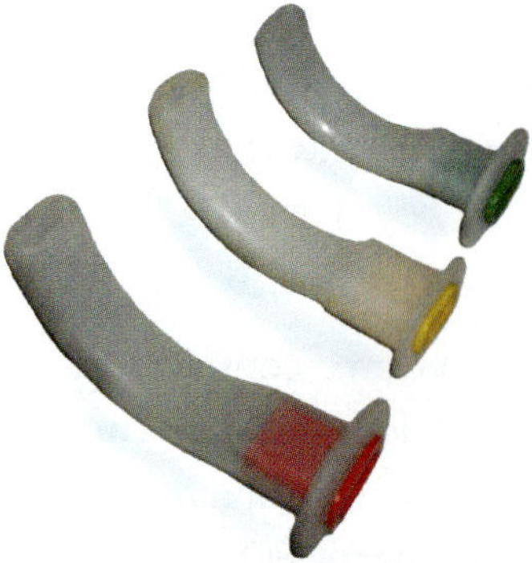

Fig. 5.1B: Airways

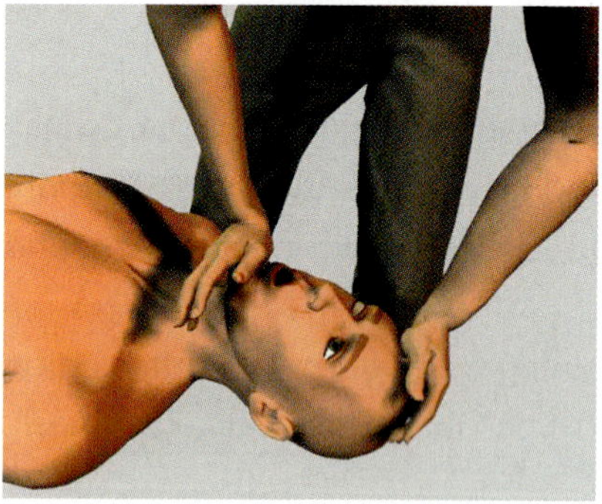

Fig. 5.1C: Airway clearance

If the patient's airway is free but breathing is not present or insufficient, then insert an airway, and ventilate with Ambubag and 100% oxygen (If Ambubag is not available, use expired air ventilation, consisting of mouth-to-mouth breathing technique). This should be continued till the patient is brought to the hospital (Figs 5.2A to C).

Ambubag ventilation is done at a rate of 15 – 20 per minute.

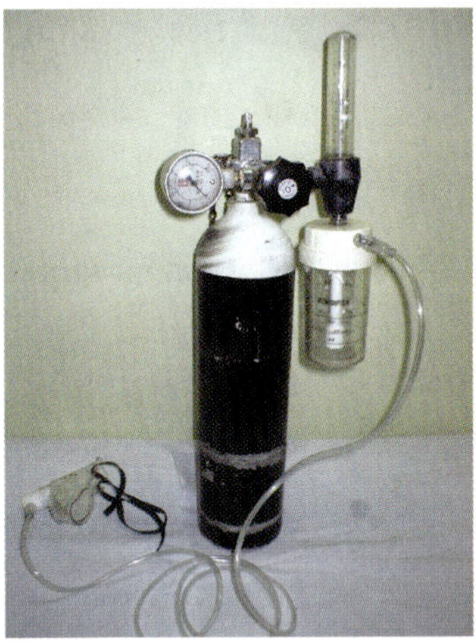

Fig. 5.2A: Oxygen cylinder equipment

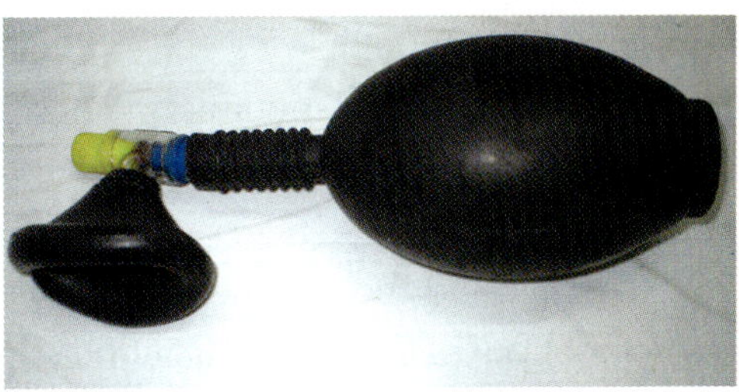

Fig. 5.2B: Ambubag

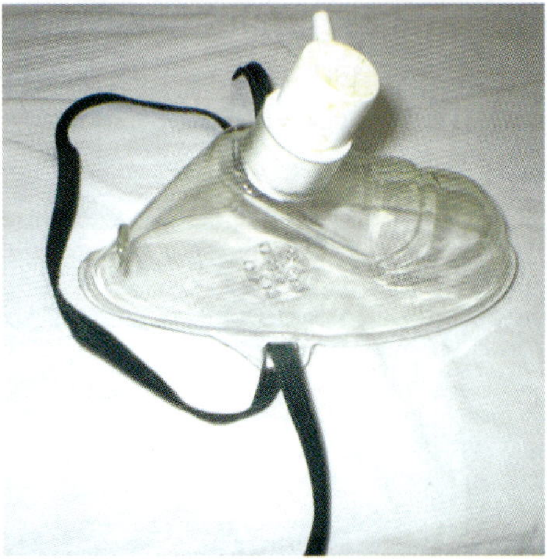

Fig. 5.2C: Face mask

Mouth-to-Mouth Breathing

1. Kneel beside the victim. Tilt the head back and keep the airway open.
2. Close the nose by pinching it with thumb and index fingers.
3. Take a deep breath. Put your open mouth over the victims open mouth making a tight seal with your lips around the victim's mouth.
4. Breath out into the victim's mouth and check that the victim's chest rising up. The breath should last for 2 seconds.
5. Lift your head up and see the chest of the victim falls as the air comes out of the airway. Continue the rescue breathing for 5 times.

6. Check for signs of circulation. If there is no circulation, do CPR. If there is circulation, continue rescue breathing till the patient is brought to a hospital.

Once the victim starts spontaneous breathing, turn the victim on to the side into the recovery position (Figs 5.3A to F).

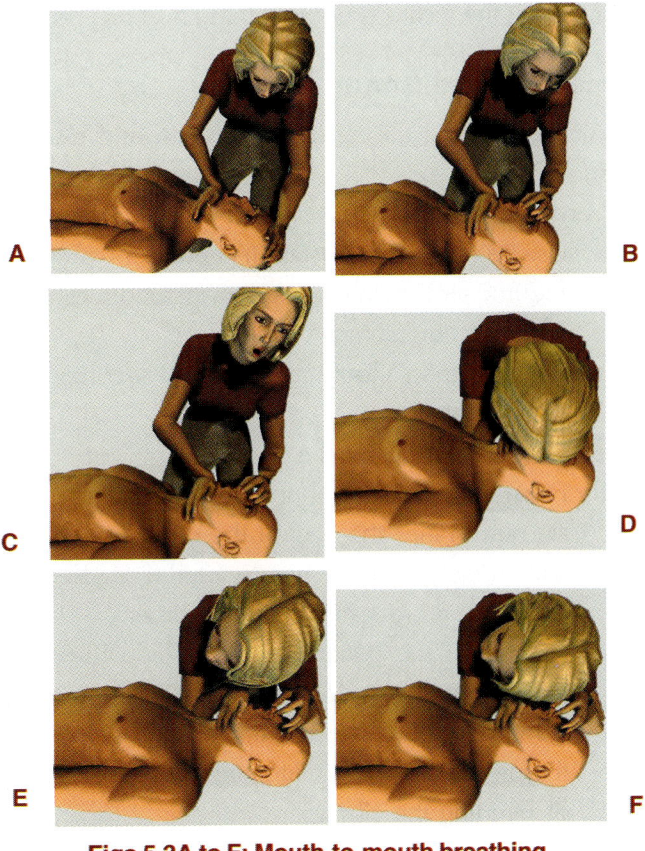

Figs 5.3A to F: Mouth-to-mouth breathing

CPR (CARDIOPULMONARY RESUSCITATION)

CPR is the technique of providing basic life support using chest compression and artificial ventilation. CPR is required after a cardiac arrest, when the heart has stopped beating resulting in stagnation of circulation.

CPR should be started immediately as soon as it is noticed that the victim is not breathing and has no pulse.

Procedure (Figs 5.4A to D)

1. Airway: Extend the neck, lift the chin and clean the mouth.
2. Ventilation:
   a. Use bag and mask system (Ambubag) – preferable
   b. Expired air ventilation – with mask or direct mouth-to-mouth breathing.
   c. Each inflation should take about 2 seconds.
3. Chest compression
   a. Kneel down beside the patient
   b. Place the heel of one hand over the lower 1/3rd of sternum. Place the heel of the other hand on top with fingers of both hands interlaced. Keep the elbows and arms straight all the time.
   c. Lean over the patient so as to keep the hands, elbows and shoulders in one line vertically. Compress the chest wall down by 5 cm. Release the pressure without taking the hands of the chest or bending the elbows.

d. Aim for 5 cm. Compressions at 100 per minute.

If alone, give 15 compressions to 2 breaths (15:2)

If 2 persons are present, give 5 compressions to 1 breath (5:1).

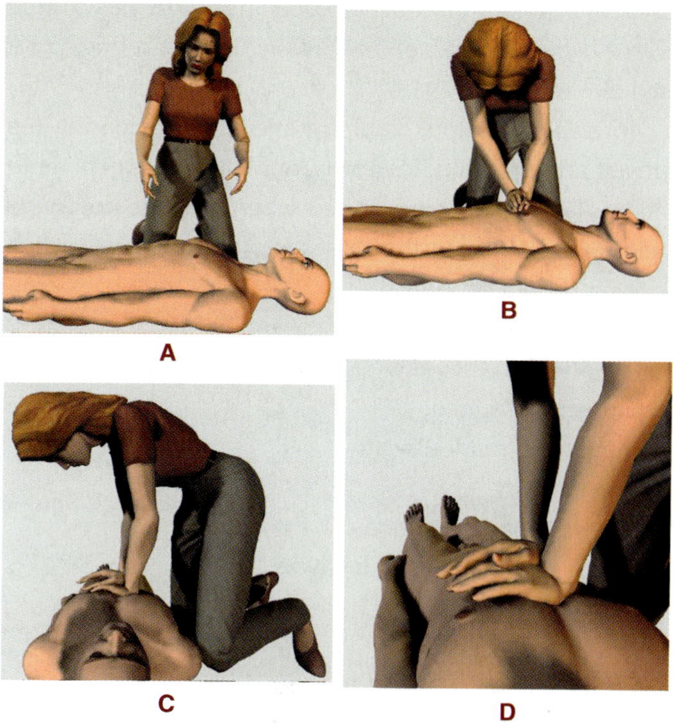

Figs 5.4A to D: Cardiopulmonary resuscitation

CPR should not be interrupted except to give defibrillator shocks or for introduction of laryngeal mask airway (LMA). Continue CPR till the patient is taken to the hospital.

LARYNGEAL MASK AIRWAY (LMA)

LMA is the technique of securing an airway by inserting a Laryngeal Mask Airway on to the Larynx. This is a safe and blind insertion which means a Laryngoscope is not used to visualize the tracheal opening. LMA has a tube with a cuffed (inflatable) mask at the distal end (Figs 5.5A and B).

In an unconscious trauma patient, after clearing the airway and inserting an airway, and giving oxygen ventilation, then LMA is introduced when there is no cough reflex or Gag reflex by the patient as oropharyngeal suction is done (Figs 5.6A and B).

Procedure

Equipment required:
- Laryngeal mask airway
- Connectors
- Inflating bag (Ambubag)
- 10 ml syringe for cuff inflation
- Suction apparatus

Technique

- Deflate the cuff.
- Lubricate the back side of the mask with lignocaine jelly.
- Hold the LMA like a pen, with the index finger placed at the junction of the cuff and the tube.

- With the head extended, introduce the LMA in the mouth flattening the cuff against the hard palate.
- Use Index finger to push cranially in to the Pharynx. Advance the tube until definite resistance is felt.
- Remove the index finger and inflate the cuff.
- Now connect the Ambubag and start ventilation with oxygen and auscultate the chest on both sides for breath sounds.

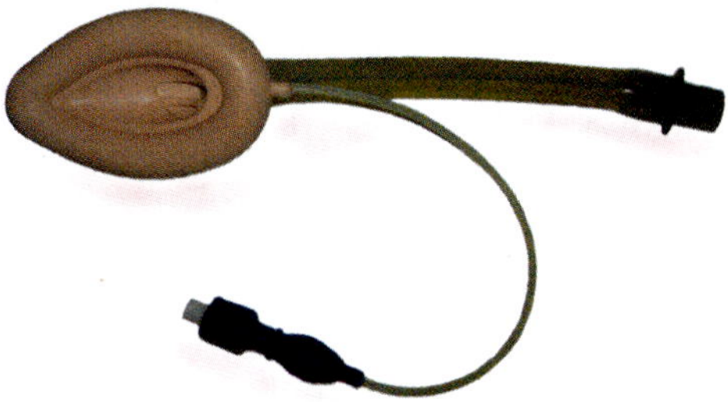

Fig. 5.5A: Laryngeal mask airway

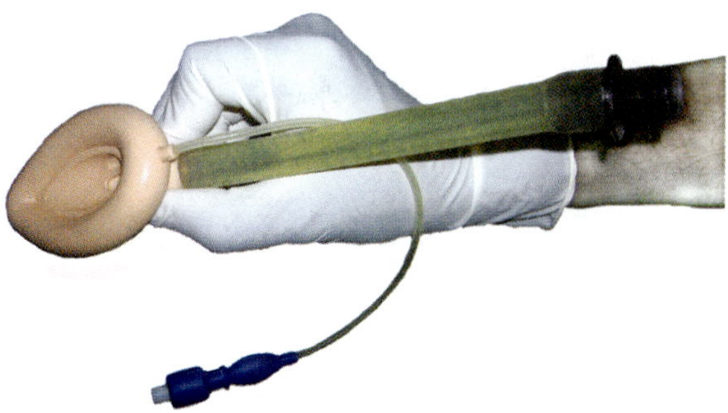

Fig. 5.5B: LMA holding

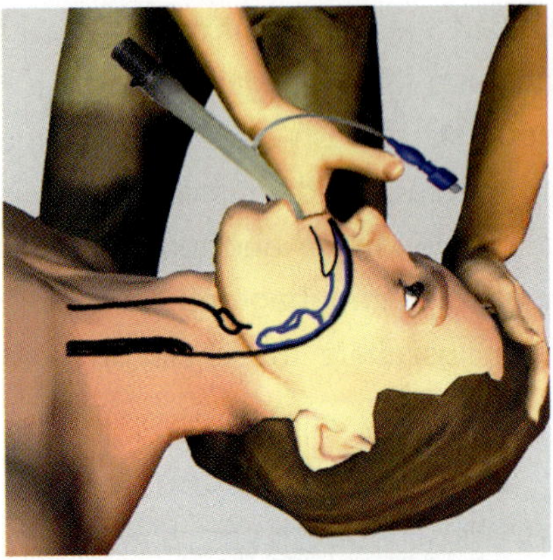

Fig. 5.6A: LMA insertion – using index finger

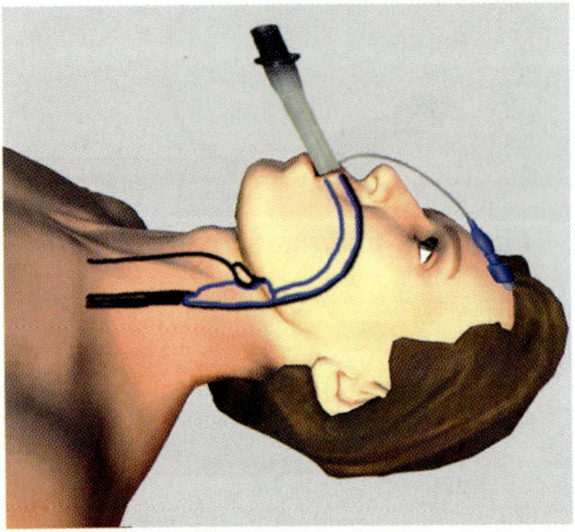

Fig. 5.6B: LMA insertion till resistance

Cautions

Cervical spine of the unconscious patient should be considered broken and proper care of the neck should be taken throughout the procedure. This involves not to move the neck but to stabilize the neck without traction (by using a spine board, sand bags, or a hard collar).

IV FLUID TRANSFUSION

Intravenous fluids are very important to save the lives of trauma patients who have lost blood or nutrients. Actually blood replacement is ideal but blood cannot be made available readily at the site of the accident, so fluid replacement is necessary.

Intravenous-Cannula (Intracath) Insertion (Fig. 5.7)

Site: Peripheral veins in the non-injured limb should be selected. In case of upper limb, select the veins on the back of hand or in front of the elbow. In case of lower limb, select the veins on the foot or on the inner side of ankle.

Install two or more lines depending on the severity of the injury.

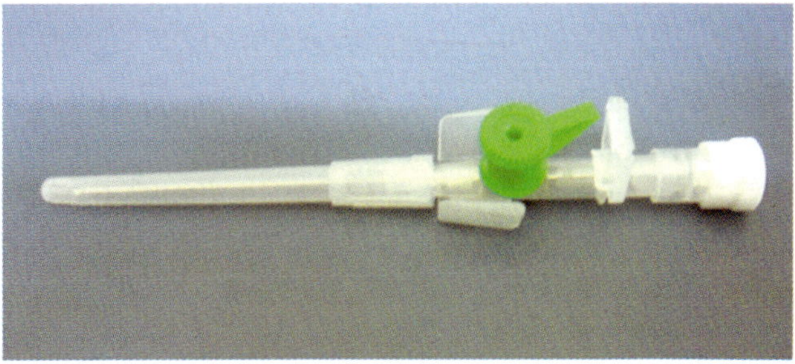

Fig. 5.7: Intracath

Technique (Fig. 5.8)

Use a 14 or 16 gauge needle. First apply the Tourniquet band to the upper-arm (thigh for lower limb) to fill up the veins. Clean the skin over the selected vein site with spirit swab. Open the Intracath package, hold the Intracath with the folded flaps and remove the cap over the needle. With the needle touching the skin at an angle of less than 45 degrees, push the needle in to the skin over the vein. Slowly push the needle on the vein. As you penetrate the vein, blood flows around the shaft of the needle. Now reduce the angle and slowly withdraw the stylus (needle) with one hand while holding the flaps with other hand. As the stylus is being withdrawn you should see the blood filling in the sleeve beyond the tip of the needle. Now advance the sleeve further in the vein. Secure the Intracath with adhesive tape after unfolding the flaps. Remove the needle completely and connect the tube from the IV-set.

IV Fluids

First start with a crystalloid solution like Ringer lactate or DNS.

If the blood loss is more, start another side Intracath and use Colloid solution like Hemaccel.

In case of a patient in shock, make sure that fluids are running in very fast. Continue IV fluids till the patient is brought to the hospital.

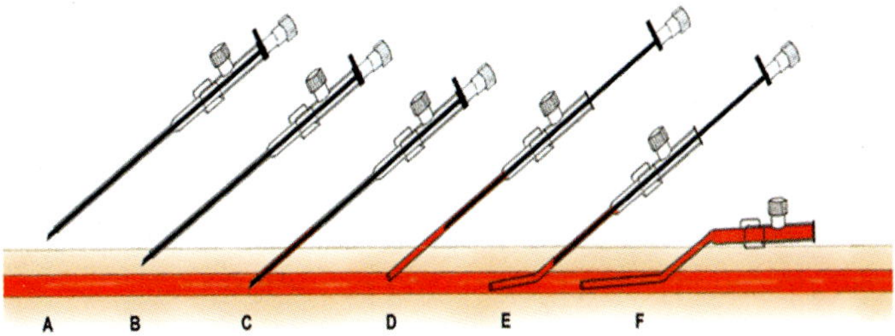

Fig. 5.8: Intracath insertion: A. Tip on the skin B. Skin penetration C. Vessel penetration D. Withdraw stylus partly E. Advance cannula F. Stylus removal

STOPPING BLEEDING

Any bleeding can be controlled with local pressure. Abdominal and chest wound bleeding is difficult to control at the site of accident. Keep a sterile dressing and apply a firm pressure.

Limb injury bleeding can be controlled by elevation of the injured limb and by applying firm pressure with a pad or fingers. Once the bleeding is stopped, apply a sterile dressing and bandage over the wound.

Tourniquet is rarely used.

CARE OF NECK AND SPINE

Any trauma patient who is not fully conscious, should be assumed to be having an injury of the neck or back until proved otherwise.

ABC, Spinal Board, Hard Collar

The care of the airway is a priority, but in almost all cases this can be managed with due care of the spine. Manual spinal protection should be instituted immediately. The application of definitive immobilization devices should not take precedence over life-saving procedures.

If the neck is not in the neutral position, an attempt should be made to achieve alignment. If the patient is awake and co-operative, they should actively move their neck into line. If unconscious or unable to co-operate this is done passively. If there is any pain, neurological deterioration or resistance to movement the procedure should be abandoned and the neck splinted in the current position (Fig. 5.9).

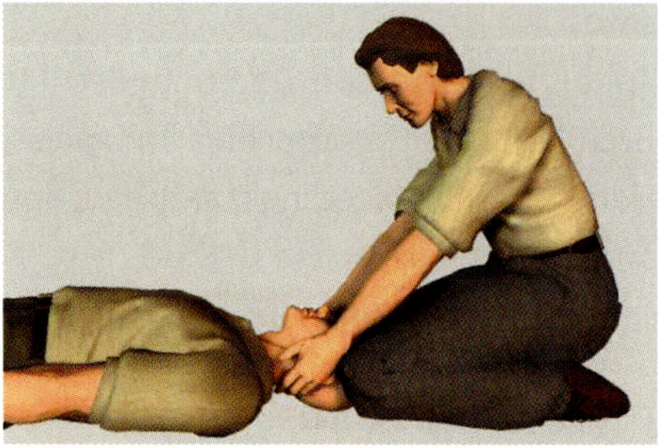

Fig. 5.9: Care of neck

Techniques of Immobilization and Patient Handling

The spine should be protected at all times during the management of the multiply injured patient. The ideal position is with the whole spine immobilized in a neutral position on a firm surface. This may be achieved manually or with a combination of semi-rigid cervical collar, side head supports and strapping. Strapping should be applied to the shoulders and pelvis as well as the head to prevent the neck becoming the center of rotation of the body (Figs 5.10A and B).

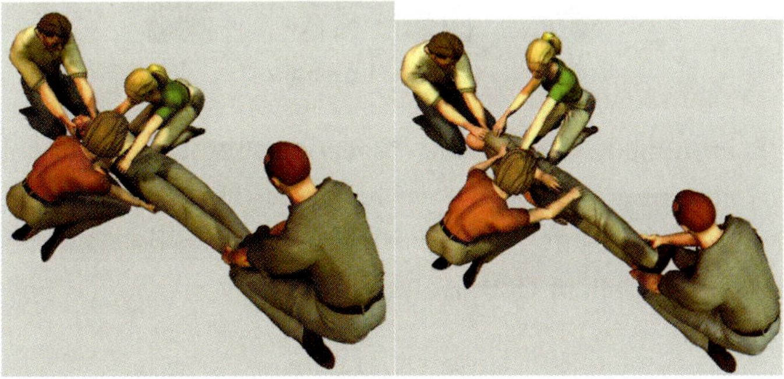

A B

Figs 5.10A and B: Log roll

The log roll is the standard maneuver to allow examination of the back and transfer on and off back boards. Four to six people are required, one holding the head and coordinating the roll, and three to roll the chest, pelvis and limbs. The number and degree of rolls should be kept to an absolute minimum and should be done as a synchronized movement (Fig. 5.11).

Patients who are agitated or restless due to shock, hypoxia, head injury or intoxication may be impossible

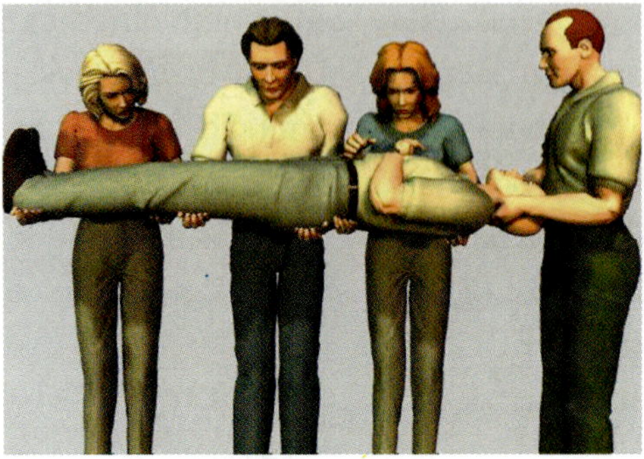

Fig. 5.11: Log lift

to immobilize adequately. Forced restraints or manual fixation of the head may risk further injury to the spine. It may be necessary to remove immobilization devices and allow the patient to move unhindered.

Chapter 6

First Aid

ANTISEPSIS

Sepsis is infection of any tissue in the body by microorganisms like Bacteria, Viruses, Fungi, etc.

A sterile material or environment is one which does not harbour or carry any living microorganisms or spores.

Surgical materials like Dressings, Instruments, Implants, etc. are made sterile by sterilizing techniques like autoclaving, gamma radiation, chemicals (CIDEX, Formalin), etc. When any sealed sterile packing is opened, the contents should be used immediately, otherwise it is considered contaminated and should be discarded or re-sterilized.

Antisepsis is the use of drugs or chemicals locally on the wound surface for curing and prevention of infection. Any open wound, specially in a road traffic accident is prone for infection if the contamination is not removed or the wound is left open for a long time. Any wound which gets infected, leads to pus formation, and can lead to septicemia (spread of infection to bloodstream) and can be fatal sometimes in spite of treatment. So, as prevention is always better than cure, any open wound should be covered immediately with sterile dressings till the patient is taken to the hospital.

Aseptic technique is the use or handling of sterile materials with minimal touching and maneuvering to prevent contamination of materials.

DRESSING MATERIALS

A standard dressing consists of 3 layers (Fig. 6.1).

First layer: This is the one which is placed on the wound surface. This is a Non-adherent layer. This is usually a piece of gauze applied directly on the wound surface. Many times this gauze is impregnated with some antibiotics like Betadine or Soframycin and with Vaseline to make it non-adherent to skin or wound surface (Products available in a drug store – Sofratulle, Bactigras, etc.).

Second layer: This is an Absorbent layer. This consists of a thick layer of cotton wool a layer of gauze on both sides, usually called GAMGI PADS. Its purpose is to absorb any ooze of blood or discharge from the wounds (Products – Steripads).

Third layer: This is the Retaining layer. Its purpose is to hold the dressing in its place and sometimes to give a mild compressive action to reduce swelling or effusion. This consists of strips of adhesive tape or gauze bandage. For compression – Crepe bandage is used (Products–Micropore Tape, Roller bandage, Crepe bandage).

WOUND CLEANING

Any wound needs to be cleaned of contamination like dirt and foreign material and any blood and secretions. Cleaning is usually done with sterile saline using sterile gloves and gauze pads.

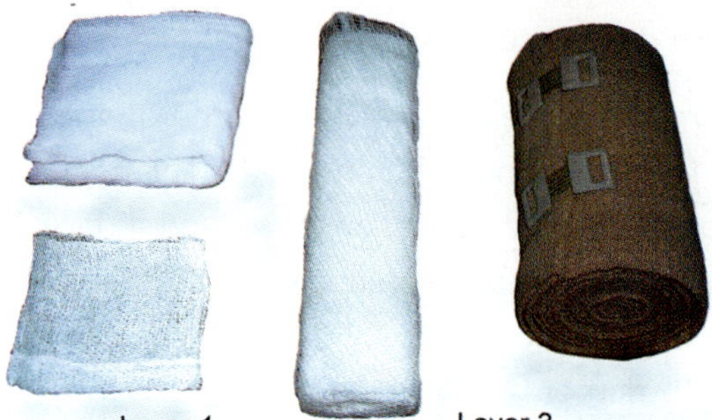

Fig. 6.1: Dressing layers

In a road accident set up, we cannot expect a thorough cleaning of the wound. One should not waste time in thorough cleaning of the wound. A minimal and gross cleaning should be done as quickly as possible.

Any superficial floating dirt and foreign material can be removed quickly by squirting saline with a syringe. But any deep penetrating object should not be removed (to be removed by a Surgeon in the OT). Any broken pieces of bone should be left intact.

DRESSING APPLICATION

The purpose of Dressing application is to cover the wound from external environment as early as possible so that the chances of wound infection is reduced. Resuscitation of patient is of prime importance and dressing application should not interfere with resuscitation unless a major bleeding needs to be stopped.

After cleaning of the wound, Betadine lotion is instilled into the wound or Betadine gauze is applied on the wound surface. Then absorbent pads applied and a loose bandage is applied with roller gauze bandage. Bandage should not be applied too tightly as it may act as a tourniquet and stop the blood flow.

In case of soakage of dressing with blood, simply put more pads on the side of the soakage and apply a bandage, without opening the dressing and wasting time.

SPLINT APPLICATION

The purpose of a Splint is to give a rigid external support to a broken or unstable part of the body so as to avoid further damage to soft tissues or arteries or nerves.

Any rigid material like wooden plank or stick, metal strips or rods, plastic strips, ruler, twigs, etc. can be used. It should be properly padded with cotton wool, cloth or any soft material to make it comfortable and to avoid pressure points on the skin which can lead to necrosis of skin (Figs 6.2A and B).

Splint should not be applied too tightly else it may act as a tourniquet and stop the blood flow. Distal pulsations should always be checked before and after application of a splint.

The length of the splint should encompass the neighboring two joints or bones for its proper effect and support. For example, in case of a fracture of leg, it should encompass the knee and ankle in the splint. In case of a knee

Figs 6.2A and B: Simple splint with three wooden planks and velcro

injury, it should enclose the upper thigh and lower leg in the splint.

After splinting, the limb should be kept elevated for proper venous drainage. In case of increased pain, discomfort or loss of pulsation, the splint should be removed immediately (Fig. 6.3).

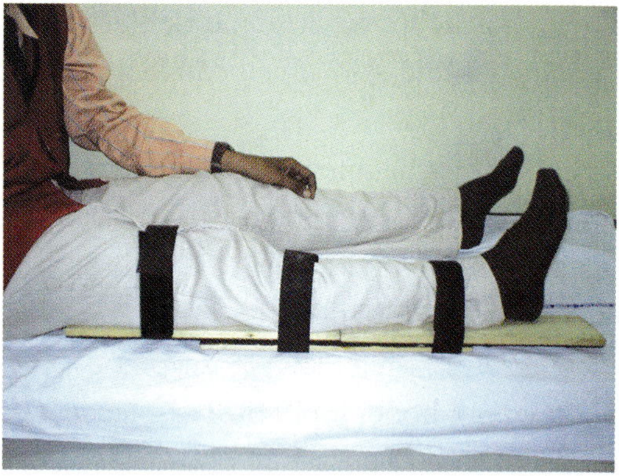

Fig. 6.3: Splint application

Chapter 7

Miscellaneous

TRANSPORTATION

The care of the trauma patient needs to be continued by the Paramedic, even after resuscitation, till the patient is brought to a hospital or trauma care center.

He/she should could co-ordinate the proper shifting of the patient from the accident site to an ambulance. Sometimes the patient may be trapped in or under a crushed vehicle and needs co-ordination with Police, Fire Brigade, etc.

The basic principle involved in good shifting and transportation of the patient is that further injury should be avoided. Any form of movement involves change of position and inertia which can be harmful. All movements should be slow and coordinated and should be kept to a minimum. All jerky and unnecessary movements of the patient should be avoided. Maximum movements occur as stretchers are man-handled into vehicles.

During the transport of the patient, in an ambulance, continuous monitoring of the patent's vitals should be done and be prepared for any resuscitative measure to be undertaken when required.

Psychology

The overriding principle, as in any medical management, is ***Primum non nocere***, that is, first do no harm.

A Paramedic is not a Doctor. He/she has capabilities and limitations to work with. At times the paramedic may be the only person to save the life of a trauma victim at the site of the accident. The paramedic needs to quickly assess the patient and act promptly by resuscitating the patient. This requires "First-Hour Competence" to save lives, reduce morbidity and avoid unnecessary harm. At other times, the paramedic may be assisting a skilled doctor in resuscitating the patient.

A paramedic should wear a uniform and display an ID card and carry the emergency kit. The paramedic should practice the skills listed in the Appendix 2 on a daily basis to maintain the First-Hour Competence. He/she should maintain the emergency kit properly. He/she should maintain coolness and poise and show compassion while caring for the patient and to get agitated at the accident site.

A paramedic, though not a doctor, may be legally bound for malpractice in case of negligence.

Documentation

Documentation of the trauma patient is very important. But the first priority is resuscitation and care of the patient. Documentation can be done during the transfer of the patient or after arrival of the patent at a Trauma center or hospital.

The following details need to be recorded:

A. Details about the accident
   - Site
   - Time
   - Description of the accident

B. Details about the patient

- Initial status/assessment and time
- Resuscitation measures
- Response to resuscitation
- Other measures – Splints, First Aid
- Transportation

Appendices

ALGORITHM

Trauma Algorithm—Global Hospitals

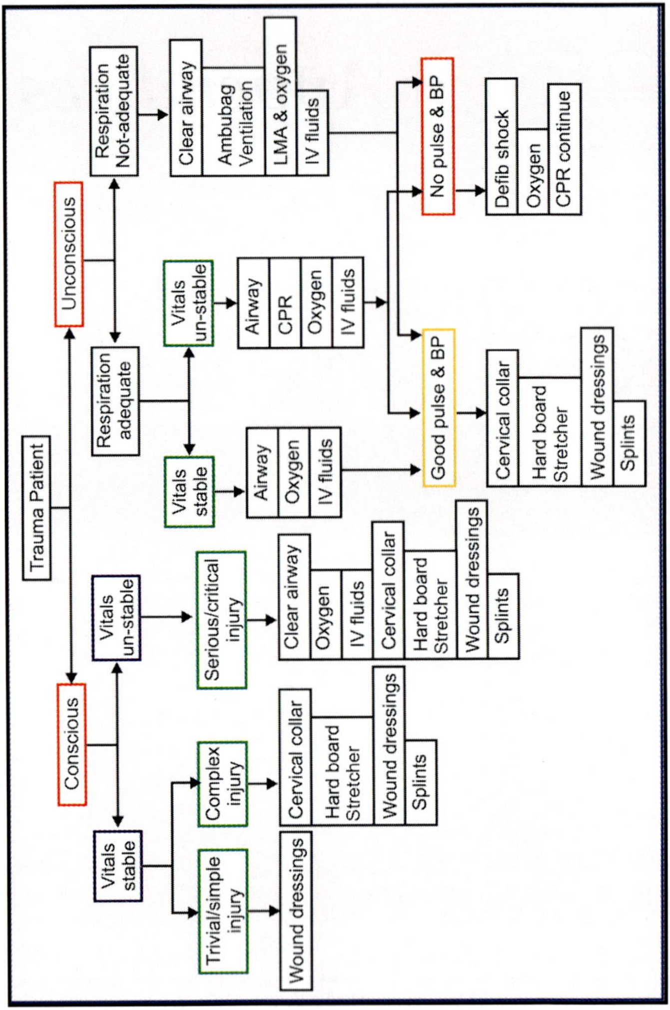

TWO WHEELER PARAMEDIC KIT

S. No	*Items*	*Quantity*
1	Airway	1
2	Oxygen mask	1
3	Oxygen cylinder	1
4	Ambubag	1
5	Intracath 18 & 20 G	1 each
6	IV Sets	2
7	IV fluids RL	2
8	Dressing tray	1
9	Betadine solution	1
10	Bandages 6" & 4"	1 pack each
11	Splints	1
12	Syringes 2 and 5 ml	5 each
13	Gloves	5 pairs
14	Torch and batteries	1
15	Scissors	1 pair
16	Tongue depressors	3
17	Adhesive tape 1"	1
18	LMA	1
19	Hand sucker	1

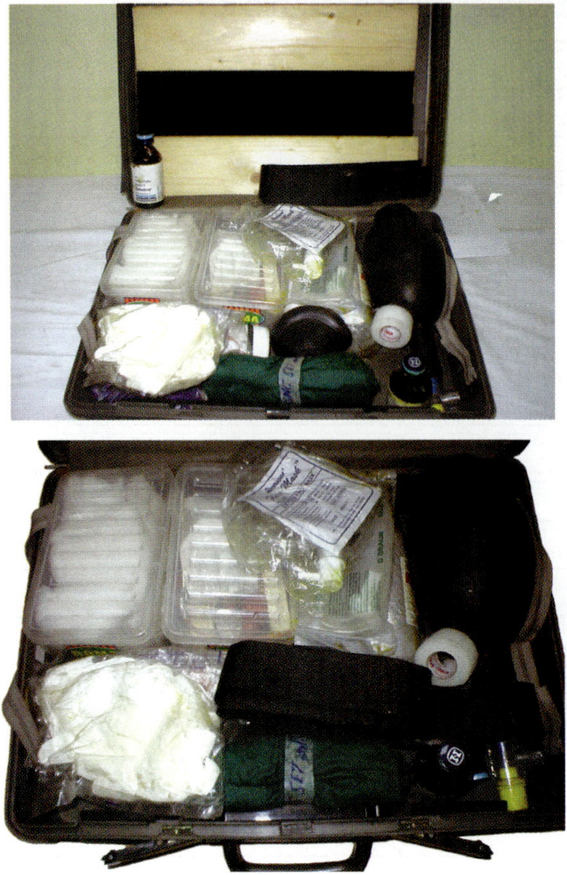

Fig. A1: Paramedic kit of G-ART

PARAMEDIC DAILY EXERCISES

S. No	*Topic*	*Items*	*Notes*
A.	Approaching the Patient	Not to panic Quick action	
B.	Clinical methods—Assessment	Consciousness Pulse BP Auscultation Temperature Pulse oxymeter	
C.	Clinical methods—Actions	Injections IM / IV IV fluids Airway clearance Oxygen inhalation Ambubag ventilation CPR Cervical collar Hard board Stretcher Wound dressings Splints application	
D.	Maintenance of Equipment	Check all items	

PARAMEDIC TRAINING TIME-TABLE

S. No	Week	Day	Topic	Lecturer	Notes
	1st		**Human Anatomy & Physiology**		
1		1	Respiratory system		
2		2	Circulatory system		
3		3	G-I System & urinary system		
4		4	Nervous system		
5		5	Musculo-skeletal system		
6		6	Simple clinical methods		
	2nd		**Injury & Dynamics**		
7		1	Types of Injuries		
8		2	Shock		
9		3	Head injury		
10		4	Face injury		
11		5	Chest injury		
12		6	Abdomen injury		
13	**3rd**	1	Urinary Injury		
14		2	Neck & back injury		
15		3	Limb injury		
16		4	Burn injury		
			Patient Evaluation		
17		5	Consciousness & respiration		
18		6	Pulse, BP & heart sounds		
19	**4th**	1	Bleeding & Vomiting		
20		2	Sit, Stand & Walk & Limb movements		
			Resuscitation		
21		3	ABCD		
22		4	Airway clearance		
23		5	Oxygen inhalation & ventilation		
24		6	CPR		

Contd...

25	**5th**	1	LMA
26		2	IV fluid transfusion
27		3	Stop bleeding
28		4	Care of neck & spine
			First Aid
29		5	Antisepsis & dressing materials
30		6	Wound cleaning & dressing application
31	**6th**	1	Splint Application
			Patient Transportation, Psychology & Documentation
32		2	Transportation & psychology
33		3	Documentation
			Evaluation & Counseling
34		4	Examination
35		5	Counseling
36		6	Celebration

MCQs

PART—A

1. You see an accident victim lying on the road. What do you do first?

A. Call for help
B. Call for police
C. Check airway

2. You see an accident victim lying on the road. To know whether the person is conscious or not what do you do?

A. Check BP
B. Check breathing
C. Ask questions

3. An unconscious accident victim is lying on the road. Breathing is good and BP is stable. What do you suspect?

A. Chest injury
B. Head injury
C. Abdominal injury

4. A conscious person lying on the road. He is not able to move any limb. What do you suspect?

A. Broken limbs
B. Shock
C. Cervical spine injury

5. You see an accident victim lying on the road. Pulse is not palpable and breathing is absent. What do you do?

A. CPR
B. Call for Ambulance
C. Try to wake up the patient

6. **You see an accident victim lying on the road. Pulse is weak and fast and no breathing. What do you do?**

   A. CPR
   B. Mouth-to-mouth breathing
   C. Start IV fluids

7. **You see an accident victim lying on the road. Breathing is present but pulse is fast and weak with BP of 90/50 mm of Hg. What do you do first?**

   A. CPR
   B. IV fluids
   C. Elevate the feet

8. **8. You see an accident victim lying on the road. Breathing is present but pulse is fast and weak with BP of 90/50 mm of Hg. What do you do?**

   A. CPR
   B. IV fluids
   C. Make the person sit up

9. **You see an accident victim lying on the road. Breathing well, Pulse is 120 per minute, BP is 90/50 mm of Hg. He wants to drink water. What do you do?**

   A. Give him water for drinking
   B. Start IV fluids
   C. Give oxygen inhalation

10. **You see an unconscious accident victim lying on the road. Airway is clear. Breathing well, Pulse and BP are normal. What do you do first?**

    A. Give oxygen inhalation
    B. Do CPR
    C. Insert an airway

11. You see an unconscious accident victim lying on the road with head injury. Airway is clear, Breathing, Pulse and BP are OK. What do you do?

A. IV fluids
B. Oxygen inhalation
C. Wake up the patient

12. You see an accident victim lying on the road with severe injury to face and mouth. What do you do first?

A. Oxygen inhalation
B. IV fluids
C. Airway clearance

13. You see an accident victim lying on the road with open chest injury and difficulty in breathing. What do you do first?

A. Oxygen inhalation
B. IV fluids
C. Cover the wound with dressing

14. You see an accident victim lying on the road with open chest injury and difficulty in breathing. What do you do?

A. IV fluids
B. Intubation and ventilation
C. Chest compressions

15. You see an accident victim lying on the road with open chest injury and no breathing and pulse. What do you do?

A. Oxygen inhalation
B. CPR
C. IV fluids

16. You need to transport a patient with spine injury. Which one do you choose?

A. Sitting in comfortable position
B. Semi-sitting and to one side
C. Supine – rigid board

17. You see an accident victim lying on the road with open injury of the abdomen. Breathing well, Pulse is 110 per minute and BP is 110/60 mm of Hg. What do you do?

A. IV fluids
B. Dressing of the wound
C. Oxygen inhalation

18. You see an accident victim lying on the road with a pulsating bleeding from the wound in the arm. What do you do first?

A. IV fluids
B. Pressure application to stop bleeding
C. Oxygen inhalation

19. You see an accident victim lying on the road with inability to move both the lower limbs. What do you suspect?

A. Head injury
B. Spine injury
C. Fracture of both lower limbs

20. You are alone doing CPR on a patient. How many chest compressions to breathing do you do?

A. 10 : 2
B. 15 : 2
C. 20 : 2

PART—B

1. Who is a Paramedic?

A. A person sitting by the side of a medical doctor
B. A person who can handle all medical problems
C. A person who can initiate medical emergency care

2. What is normal pulse rate?

A. 60 per minute
B. 72 per minute
C. 80 per minute

3. How do you know easily that a patient is breathing or not?

A. By chest movements
B. By abdomen movements
C. By feeling of air flow on the back of fingers kept close to nose

4. What is normal respiratory rate?

A. 10 per minute
B. 20 per minute
C. 30 per minute

5. What is normal blood pressure?

A. 80/60 mm of Hg
B. 120/80 mm of Hg
C. 150/90 mm of Hg

6. What do you think if blood pressure is 60/40 mm of Hg in an accident patient?

A. It is normal
B. It is low and needs IV fluids immediately
C. You can wait till the patient reaches hospital

7. What do you think if blood pressure is 150/100 mm of Hg in accident patient?

- **A.** It is high and may have head injury and needs Neurosurgical referral
- **B.** It can be normal and nothing to be done
- **C.** It is high and needs IV fluids

8. In a trauma case if pulse rate is more than 100 per minute, what do you think?

- **A.** It is high and needs analgesic to subside
- **B.** It is high and needs IV fluids immediately
- **C.** It is high and needs to be referred to neighboring hospital

9. Multiple injured patient on road side needs?

- **A.** Cardiac massage or CPR
- **B.** Defibrillator shock
- **C.** Wide bore needle IV fluids and referral

10. In the management of trauma victim the following is considered first:

- **A.** Circulation
- **B.** Breathing
- **C.** Airway

11. Good results can be achieved in trauma management

- **A.** If treatment starts within first hour
- **B.** If treatment is started after 3 hours
- **C.** If treatment is started after 6 hours

12. Neck should be stabilized

- **A.** To improve breathing
- **B.** To prevent further damage to spinal cord
- **C.** To prevent vomiting

13. Injuries should be assessed Primarily for:

A. Evaluation of blood loss
B. Documentation
C. To inform police

14. Vomiting can be a sign of:

A. Chest injury
B. Neck injury
C. Head injury

15. In a trauma patient with breathing problem:

A. Clear the upper airway by finger and or suction
B. Tear off the clothes
C. Put oxygen mask blindly

16. Concentration of oxygen in atmosphere air:

A. 20%
B. 30%
C. 50%

17. Cardiovascular system in the body:

A. Has water supplying electrolytes to all parts of body
B. Has lymph to supply nutrients to the whole body
C. Has blood to supply oxygen and nutrients to whole body

18. What is golden hour in trauma cases:

A. Peak traffic hour when most accidents take place
B. First hour after injury to start resuscitation
C. Safe hour to transfer the patient to a hospital

19. Endo-tracheal Intubation or LMA is necessary:

A. When there is no respiratory effort
B. When there is slowing of respiration
C. When there is rapid respiration

20. One pupil dilatation in an injured patient signifies:

- **A.** Head injury with hemorrhage in brain
- **B.** Foreign body in that eye
- **C.** Not significant

PART—C

1. In a case of Internal hemorrhage the patient usually has:

A. Decreased chest movements
B. Rapid and thready pulse
C. Unconscious

2. The main purpose of the Paramedic at the site of the accident is:

A. For administrative purpose
B. For rendering initial treatment in the golden hour
C. For referring the patients to other hospitals

3. Helmet is useful:

A. For neck stabilization and prevent head injury
B. To prevent head injury
C. To prevent eye injuries

4. External blood loss can be assessed by:

A. Presence of blood on clothes and ground
B. By the size and nature of injury
C. Both

5. Oxygen is absorbed into blood:

A. By circulation of blood in heart
B. By circulation of blood in alveoli
C. By circulation of blood in upper respiratory tract

6. Oxygen is combined with hemoglobin present in:

A. White blood cells
B. Platelets
C. Red blood cells

7. **Total quantity of circulating blood present in adult:**
   - A. Three liters
   - B. Four liters
   - C. Five liters

8. **Respiratory system consists of:**
   - A. Blood vessels
   - B. Alveoli
   - C. Both

9. **In trauma patient, how much blood loss can be dangerous?**
   - A. One liter
   - B. Two liters
   - C. Three liters

10. **Contusion wound needs?**
    - A. Pressure bandage
    - B. Crushed ice pack
    - C. IV fluids

11. **Sprain is a condition where there is damage to:**
    - A. Vessels
    - B. Nerves
    - C. Ligaments

12. **In fracture spine, spinal stabilization is necessary:**
    - A. To prevent shock
    - B. To prevent hemorrhage
    - C. To prevent further damage to the spinal cord

13. **Fracture of spine is always associated with:**
    - A. Spinal cord injury
    - B. Bladder disturbance
    - C. Severe pain in the back

14. In severe burns, the instant treatment would be:

A. Cover with blankets
B. Immediate infusion with IV fluids
C. Antibiotics

15. Immediate treatment of small and simple burns:

A. Clean with cold water and pain relief tablets
B. IV fluids
C. Skin grafting

16. A driver with the seat belt injury on abdomen:

A. Suspect only outside injury
B. Suspect internal injury
C. Suspect nothing

17. A man found on the road with an abrasion above the right eyebrow:

A. Needs only a dressing
B. Needs to be seen by a doctor
C. Needs to be seen by a neurosurgeon

18. Injuries over the abdomen usually cause:

A. Internal bleeding
B. External bleeding
C. None of the above

19. You apply a cervical collar to an unconscious patient on the road because:

A. It is comfortable
B. You suspect neck injury
C. You can apply traction easily

20. A patient has an amputation of right thumb. Before taking to hospital, the best you do:

A. Put the amputated thumb on the wound (hand) and do dressing
B. Do the dressing of the amputated thumb separately
C. Put the amputated thumb in a saline bag and put the bag in an ice bag.

ANSWERS

Part—A		Part—B		Part—C	
1	C	1	C	1	B
2	C	2	B	2	B
3	B	3	C	3	B
4	C	4	B	4	C
5	A	5	B	5	B
6	B	6	B	6	C
7	C	7	A	7	C
8	B	8	B	8	C
9	B	9	C	9	A
10	C	10	C	10	B
11	B	11	A	11	C
12	C	12	B	12	C
13	C	13	A	13	C
14	B	14	C	14	A
15	B	15	A	15	A
16	C	16	A	16	B
17	A	17	C	17	C
18	B	18	B	18	A
19	B	19	A	19	B
20	A	20	A	20	C

Bibliography

1. ABC of Major Trauma by David Skinner, Peter Driscoll and Richard Earlam.
2. ATLS – Advanced Trauma Life Support by American College of Surgeons Committee on Trauma.
3. Bureau of Labor Statistics – www.bls.gov
4. First Aid Book
5. Gray's Anatomy
6. Hutchison's Clinical Methods
7. NAEMSE'S EMS BOOKS.COM
8. National Association of Emergency Medical Technicians – www.naert.org
9. National Registry of Emergency Medical Technicians – www.nrert.org
10. Virtual Naval Hospital – www.vnh.org
11. www.trauma.org